MASTERING BIOSTATISTICS AND EPIDEMIOLOGY

A Guide for USMLE Success and Beyond

Over 100 sample MCQs
with explanation and
240 exercise MCQs

SYED MOHAMED ALJUNID
YIN NWE AUNG

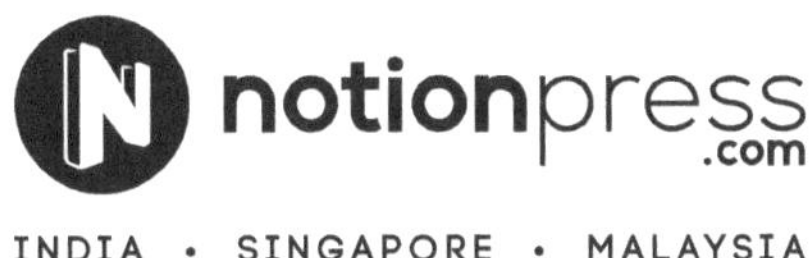

INDIA · SINGAPORE · MALAYSIA

ISBN 979-8-89699-773-3

CONTENTS

PREFACE

Biostatistics and epidemiology are fundamental to modern medicine, shaping research, clinical practice, and public health decision-making. Yet, for many undergraduate students and young doctors, these fields can appear complex and difficult to grasp. This book seeks to simplify these subjects, offering a practical and approachable guide to the key concepts that form the foundation of biostatistics and epidemiology.

Focusing on building a strong theoretical base, the book covers essential topics such as epidemiological measures, study designs, data analysis, and statistical tests. It goes beyond just teaching the basics by providing insights into how these concepts are applied in real-world clinical and research settings.

What makes this book unique is its emphasis on active learning through practical examples. Each chapter includes USMLE-style questions that closely resemble those encountered on exams. Each question is accompanied by a detailed explanation, breaking down the reasoning and analytical steps required to arrive at the correct answer. This method ensures that readers don't merely memorize facts but develop the ability to think critically and apply their knowledge effectively.

To further reinforce understanding, 240 additional exercise questions are provided at the end of the book, offering an opportunity for deeper practice and helping to build confidence. These exercises are designed to challenge and solidify the principles discussed, allowing readers to test their comprehension and prepare for their exams.

Whether you're an undergraduate just beginning your medical journey or a young doctor gearing up for the USMLE or similar exams, this book is crafted to help you master biostatistics and epidemiology. It is also a valuable resource for postgraduate students embarking on early research careers, guiding them in appraising and interpreting scientific papers. Through this guide, we hope you will not only overcome the challenges of these subjects but also recognize their importance in enhancing patient care and public health.

Welcome to your journey in mastering biostatistics and epidemiology. We wish you success as you delve into the science that underlies the practice of medicine.

Y.N.A

S.M.A

INTRODUCTION TO STATISTICS

This introductory chapter will cover basic statistical terminology and delve into measurement scales, data distribution, and their applications in statistics.

LEARNING OUTCOME:

1. Calculate the measure of central tendency (mean, median, mode).
2. Explain the effect of skewed distribution on mean, median, mode.
3. Estimate the area under the normal distribution curve.
4. Compute 95% confidence interval estimates.
5. Select an appropriate descriptive measure.

Statistics is the science and art of dealing with variation in data through collection, classification, and analysis in such a way as to obtain realistic results (Last, 1983, p100).

1.1 PARAMETERS AND STATISTICS

The population refers to the entire set of observations, patients, entities, measurements, and so on, about which we aim to draw conclusions. A sample population is a subset of this broader population, while the target population is the specific group to which we intend to generalize our conclusions. Numerical characteristics of population is known as **parameters** and that of sample is **statistics.**

1.2 VARIABLE

A variable refers to the characteristics, attributes, or qualities that we are interested in studying to draw inferences and conclusions. The term "variable" is used because its values may change depending on related factors.

1.2.1 Types of Variables

Variables are classified into independent, dependent, and confounding variables. The independent variable is expected to influence the outcome, known as the dependent variable. Confounding variables are factors that can distort the relationship between the independent and dependent variables.

1.2.2 Measurement Scales for Variables

Variables are typically measured using four different types of scales:

A) **Nominal Scale**: This scale uses a limited number of categories (names, numbers, or symbols) that cannot be ordered in any particular way. Examples include race, religion, gender, blood type, and color.

B) **Ordinal Scale**: This scale also uses a limited number of categories, but these can be ranked or ordered. Examples include cancer staging and patient severity levels.

C) **Interval Scale**: This scale features an unlimited number of equally spaced categories but does not have a true zero point. An example is temperature (Celsius).

D) **Ratio Scale**: This scale includes measurements that start from a true zero point and have equal intervals. Examples include height and weight.

1.3 DESCRIPTION OF DATA

Measures of central tendency and measures of dispersion are the most commonly used tools in descriptive statistics.

1.3.1 Measures of Central Tendency

These include statistics such as the mean, median, and mode, which provide insights into the center or typical value of the data.

A) **Mean**: The arithmetic average of a set of values, calculated by summing all the values and dividing by the number of values.

B) **Median**: The middle value in a dataset when the observations are arranged in ascending or descending order. If there is an even number of observations, the median is the average of the two middle values.

C) **Mode**: The value that appears most frequently in a frequency distribution.

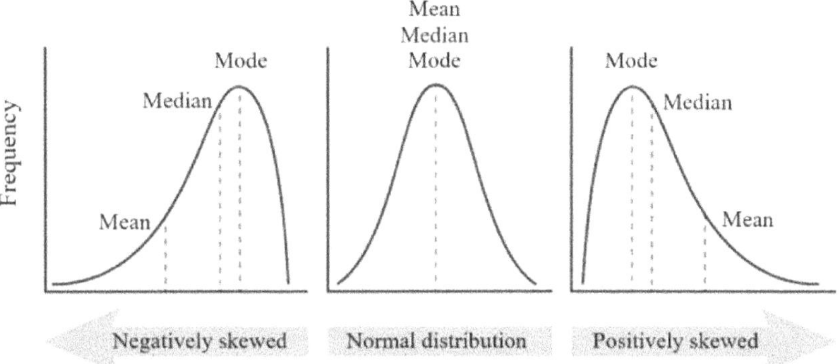

▲ **Figure 1.1:** Positioning of mean, median, mode based on distribution type

1.3.2 Measures of Dispersion

These statistics, such as range, variance, and standard deviation, describe the spread or variability of the data.

A) **Range**: Difference between the smallest and the largest numbers in a data set. It shows the spread of your data from the lowest to the highest value in the distribution.

B) **Interquartile Range (IQR):** The range of the middle 50% of the data, calculated by subtracting the first quartile (Q1) from the third quartile (Q3). It provides a measure of statistical dispersion, showing the spread of the central half of the data.

C) **Variance**: The average of the squared differences from the mean, representing how much the data points vary from the mean. The unit of variance is the square of the original unit of measurement.

  • **Population Variance**: Calculated by dividing the sum of the squared deviations by the total number of data points (n).

  • **Sample Variance**: Calculated by dividing the sum of the squared deviations by the number of data points minus one (n-1), which adjusts for the sample size.

D) **Standard Deviation**: The square root of the variance, providing a measure of the spread of the data in the same unit as the original data. It indicates how much the data points typically deviate from the mean.

E) **Standard Error:** When using samples instead of entire populations to estimate population parameters like the mean, there is inherent variability. This variability arises because the means of different samples can slightly differ from each other. This variation among sample means is calculated similarly to how the standard deviation (SD) is calculated for individual observations within a single sample. The standard deviation of the sample means is referred to as the **Standard Error (SE)** of the mean. The SE provides an estimate of how much the sample mean is expected to deviate from the true population mean.

Formula for Standard Error:

$$SE = \frac{SD}{\sqrt{n}}$$

SD: standard deviation of the sample,
n: sample size.

NB:

Difference Between Standard Deviation and Standard Error
Standard Deviation (SD):
The standard deviation measures the spread or dispersion of individual values within a data set. It indicates how much the observations in a sample vary from the sample mean. Essentially, it reflects the variability of individual data points in a normal distribution.

Standard Error of the Mean (SE):
The standard error of the mean quantifies the variability of sample means around the true population mean. It represents the degree to which the means of different samples would differ from one another. SE is crucial for estimating the true mean of the underlying population.

Effect of n, SD and SE upon CI
The magnitude of the standard error depends on both the sample size (n) and the standard deviation (SD) of the sample:

As the sample size (n) increases, SE decreases, leading to a narrower and more precise confidence interval (CI).

As the standard deviation (SD) increases, SE increases, resulting in a wider and less precise confidence interval (CI).

1.4 DISTRIBUTION OF DATA

This refers to how data points are spread out across different values and includes the shape of the data distribution. A probability distribution describes how probabilities are assigned to different outcomes of a random variable. It shows the likelihood of each outcome occurring.

There are two main types:

A) **Discrete Probability Distribution**: For variables that take on specific, countable values. Examples include the binomial and Poisson distributions.

B) **Continuous Probability Distribution**: For variables that can take any value within a range. Examples include the normal and exponential distributions.

The normal distribution is a fundamental concept in statistics. Therefore, we will concentrate solely on explaining this distribution pattern.

1.4.1 Normal Distribution

The properties of normal distribution are as follows:

A) **Bell-Shaped Curve:** The normal distribution is a continuous probability distribution characterized by a bell-shaped curve with a single peak at the mean.

B) **Symmetry Around the Mean:** One of the defining features of the normal distribution is its symmetry around the mean, allowing for easy determination of the percentage of observations within 1, 2, or 3 standard deviations (SDs).

C) **Total Area Under the Curve**: The area under the normal distribution curve represents the total probability space, which equals 1 (or 100%).

D) **68/95/99 Rule:**

- 68% of observations fall within 1 SD of the mean.
- 95% fall within 2 SDs of the mean.
- 99.7% fall within 3 SDs of the mean.

NB:

These are useful approximations, but for more precise calculation, **95%** of observations lie within **1.96 SDs** of the mean, and **99%** of observations lie within **2.58 SDs**, corresponding to specific z-scores for the normal distribution.

The values 1.96 and 2.58 are z-scores corresponding to 95% and 99% of the distribution, respectively.

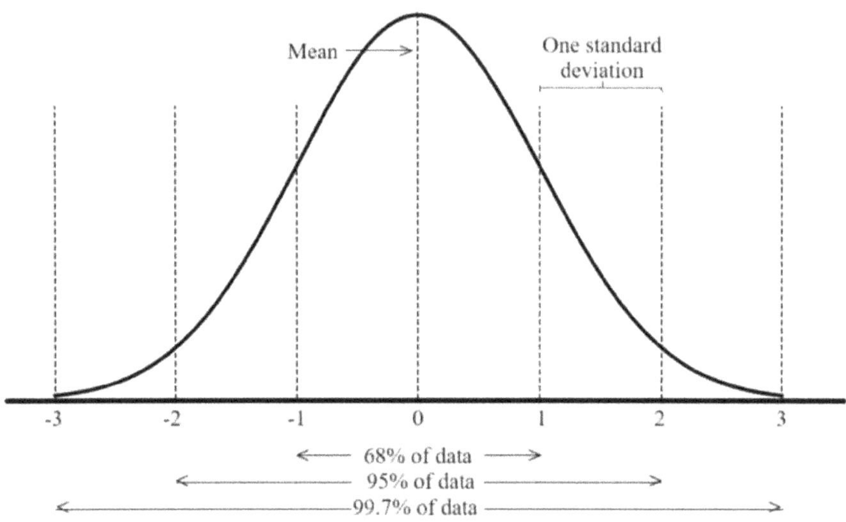

▲ **Figure 1.2:** Standard deviation of a normal distribution

1.4.2   Confidence Interval

A confidence interval (CI) helps account for this variability by incorporating the standard error (SE) into its calculation.

A 95% confidence interval provides a range within which we are 95% confident that the true population parameter (such as the mean) lies.

For example, if we calculate a 95% CI for the mean of a sample, it means that if we were to repeat the sampling process many times and calculate a confidence interval each time, approximately 95% of those intervals would contain the true population mean.

Confidence interval of mean

A sample mean provides a single estimate (point estimate) of the true population mean. However, due to the variability inherent in sampling, this estimate might not perfectly match the population mean.

Formula

CI of mean = mean± [z-score for confidence level] × SE

- For a 95% confidence level, the z-score is 1.96.

- For a 99% confidence level, the z-score is 2.58.

Thus:

- 95% CI of the mean: mean $\pm\ 1.96 \times \dfrac{SD}{\sqrt{n}}$

- 99% CI of the mean: mean $\pm\ 2.58 \times \dfrac{SD}{\sqrt{n}}$

NB:

The 95% CI does not mean there's a 95% probability that the population mean is within this specific interval; rather, it means that 95% of intervals from repeated sampling would include the population mean.

A narrower CI indicates more precision, while a wider CI suggests more variability in the estimate.

1.5   SELECTING AN APPROPRIATE DESCRIPTIVE MEASURE

Depending on the measurement scales, the findings of variables are reported in different ways.

1.5.1   Numerical Description

A) **Nominal data:** This type of data is generally described using frequency counts, percentages, or the mode. Percentages indicate the proportion of a specific category relative to the total dataset.

B) **Ordinal Data:** For data that can be ranked or ordered, descriptions often include counts, the mode, or the median. Median provides a central value that divides the data into two equal halves.

C) **Interval and Ratio Data:** When dealing with interval and ratio data, the approach depends on the distribution. For data that is normally distributed, the mean and standard deviation are used to describe the central tendency and the spread of the data, respectively. In contrast, for skewed data, the median and interquartile range (IQR) are more appropriate, as they better represent the data's central value and variability without being unduly affected by outliers.

1.5.2 Graphical Description

A) Categorical (Nominal/Ordinal) Data:

1. Pie Chart: Represents the relative proportions of categories as slices of a pie.

2. Bar Chart: Displays the frequency or proportion of categories using bars of varying lengths.

3. Stacked Bar Chart: Shows the composition of categories within a total by stacking bars on top of one another.

4. Segmented Bar Chart: Similar to stacked bars but segments within each bar represent different categories.

5. Mosaic Plot: Uses area to represent the proportion of different categories, with segments corresponding to combinations of categorical variables.

B) Continuous Data (Interval/Ratio) Data:

1. Histogram: Shows the distribution of continuous data by grouping values into bins and displaying the frequency of each bin.

2. Box Plot (Box-and-Whisker Plot): Summarizes the distribution, median, quartiles, and potential outliers of continuous data.

3. Line Graph: Used to display trends over time or a continuous variable, connecting individual data points with lines.

4. Scatter Plot: Plots individual data points on a two-dimensional graph to show the relationship between two continuous variables.

5. Density Plot: Estimates and displays the probability density function of continuous data, showing where values are concentrated.

6. Violin Plot: Combines the features of a box plot and density plot to show the distribution of continuous data and its probability density.

POSSIBLE QUESTIONS FROM THIS CHAPTER

- Calculate the mean, median and mode.
- Identify the effect of skewness upon measure of central tendency.
- Calculate probability under normal distribution.
- Calculate confidence interval.

Questions on Mean, Median and Mode, and their properties

1. The frequency of upper respiratory tract infections among children under 5 years old attending the maternal and child health clinic over the past year is recorded and presented in the following graph. What is the average number of upper respiratory tract infections per child in this sample over the course of one year?

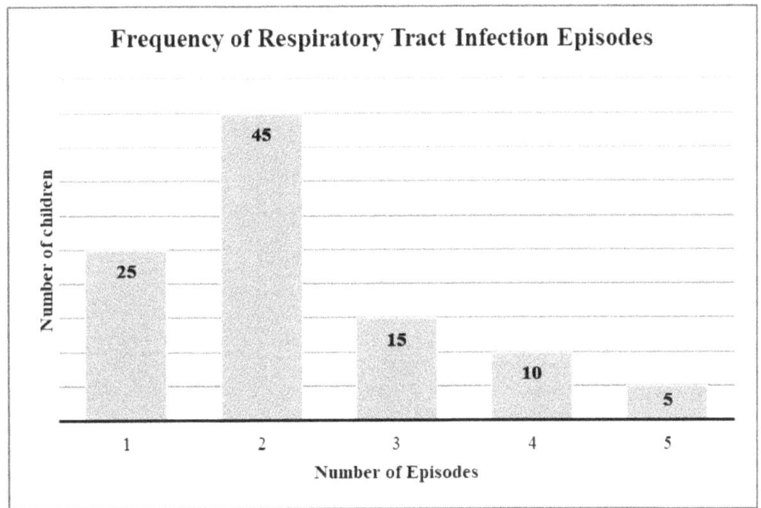

    A. Between 1 and 2

    B. 2

    C. Between 2 and 3

    D. 3

    E. Between 3 and 4

Answer: C. Between 2 and 3. $\dfrac{25+90+45+40+5}{100} = \dfrac{205}{100} = 2.05$

2. Pulmonary capillary wedge pressure (PCWP) is a useful indicator for estimating left atrial pressure, with normal values ranging from 6 to 12 mm Hg, measured in whole numbers. A patient in the intensive care unit had 7 consecutive PCWP measurements taken over a 1-hour period. The findings are as follows. 10, 8, 13, 10, 12, 16, 22. Which of the following represents the median of PCWP?

    A. 8
    B. 10
    C. 12
    D. 13
    E. 22

    Answer: C. 12. With 7 numbers in the array, the middle value is the 4th when arranged in order: 8, 10, 10, 12, 13, 16, 22. The median is 12. The mode is 10, and the mean is 13, so answers B and D are incorrect. A is the smallest value, and E is the largest value, making A and E incorrect as well.

3. A 58-year-old woman with a known history of diabetes is monitoring her fasting blood sugar (FBS) level. Consecutive readings show a minimum recorded value of 5.4 mmol/L and a maximum recorded value of 7.8 mmol/L. Her next FBS measurement is found to be 11.3 mmol/L. Which of the following is most likely to remain unchanged?

    A. Mean
    B. Mode
    C. Range
    D. Standard deviation
    E. Variance

    Answer: B. Mode. The mode is not affected by the addition of a number that was not already present in the list.

4. The hospital director reviewed patient records to determine the length of stay for admitted patients over the past year, a key indicator of hospital performance. He discovered that the data is positively skewed. Which of the following is most likely true regarding the data for the length of stay?

    A. The mean is equal to the median

    B. The mean is equal to the mode

    C. The mean is greater than the median

    D. The median is greater than the mean

    E. The mode is greater than the mean

    Answer. C. The mean is greater than the median. When a distribution is positively skewed, the mean shifts to the right, making it greater than the median.

Questions on distribution of data and standard deviation

5. A study examined hemoglobin (Hb) levels in a sample of 900 women and found the average Hb level to be 13.3 g/dL, with a standard deviation of 0.8 g/dL. Assuming the data is normally distributed, approximately 50% of the women in the sample will have Hb levels within which of the following ranges?

    A. >0 and <13.3 g/dL

    B. 11.7 to 14.9 g/dL

    C. 12.5 to 13.3 g/dL

    D. 12.5 to 14.1 g/dL

    E. <12.5 or > 14.1 g/dL

    Answer: A. > 0 and <13.3 g/dL. 50% of the population will fall below or above the median. For normally distributed data, the mean, median, and mode are the same. Thus, the median is estimated to be equivalent to the mean, which is 13.3 g/dL.

6. A study assessed serum hematocrit levels among reproductive-age women and found the mean level to be 36%, with a standard deviation of 5%. Assuming a normal distribution, approximately 95% of the hematocrit levels in this population will fall within which of the following limits?

    A. 21% to 51%

    B. 26% to 36%

    C. 26% to 46%

    D. 31% to 41%

    E. 36% to 46%

    Answer: C. 26% to 46%. Approximately 95% of the haematocrit levels will fall within mean ± 2 standard deviations (according to the empirical rule for normal distributions). Thus, 36± (2 x 5)% = 26% to 46%.

7. In a reference sample of thousands of healthy individuals, the laboratory reference range for a novel biomarker associated with liver function is 12-16 U/mL at the standard 95% confidence level. This biomarker demonstrates exceptional sensitivity and specificity for liver tissue. The hepatology team wishes to utilize a 99.7% reference range to evaluate patients presenting with elevated liver enzymes and a high pretest probability of liver disease. An elevated value for the biomarker is defined as exceeding the 99.7[th] percentile of the reference sample. Assuming a normal (Gaussian) distribution with a mean of 14 U/mL, which of the following most accurately approximates the corresponding reference range?

    A. 10.5 to 17.5 U/mL

    B. 11 to 17 U/mL

    C. 12 to 16 U/mL

    D. 13 to 15 U/mL

    E. 13.5 to 14.5 U/mL

    Answer: B. 11 to 17 U/mL. The mean is 14 U/mL with a 95% confidence interval (CI) range of 12-16 U/mL. From this information, 1 standard deviation (SD) is 1 U/mL. For 99.7% coverage, which corresponds to 3 SDs, the range becomes 14 ± 3, resulting in 11 to 17 U/mL.

8. Cholesterol levels were measured in a sample of individuals without any known health issues. The mean total cholesterol levels and corresponding standard deviations (SDs) for men and women across various age groups are presented below:

Men		Women	
Age Group	Mean Total Cholesterol (mg/dL) ± SD	Age Group	Mean Total Cholesterol (mg/dL) ± SD
35-44	190 ± 30	35-44	185 ± 25
45-54	210 ± 35	45-54	215 ± 30
55-64	230 ± 40	55-64	240 ± 35

If high cholesterol is defined as levels exceeding 245 mg/dL, what percentage of men aged 45-54 in this sample would likely be classified as having high cholesterol, assuming a normal (Gaussian) distribution?

A. 16%

B. 34%

C. 50%

D. 68%

E. 95%

Answer: A. 16%. For men aged 45-54, the average cholesterol level is 210 ± 35 mg/dL. A cholesterol level of 245 mg/dL is one standard deviation (SD) above the mean. The area within 1 SD of the mean covers 68% of the data—34% on the left side of the mean and 34% on the right side. The total area to the right of the mean is 50%. Subtracting the 34% from this, we find that 16% of men will have cholesterol levels beyond the cutoff value, indicating high cholesterol.

9. A study was conducted to examine the age of first sexual intercourse among young males in two distinct groups: those who are sexually active and those who are not.

Group	Sample Size (n)	Mean Age (years)	Standard Deviation (years)
Sexually Active	30	17.5	0.5
Not Sexually Active	25	19.1	0.9

Assuming that the age of first sexual intercourse is normally distributed, what is the probability that a randomly selected sexually active male will have his first sexual experience at age 18.5 or older?

A. 0.997

B. 0.950

C. 0.680

D. 0.050

E. 0.025

Answer: E. 0.025. The mean age of first intercourse among sexually active individuals is 17.5 ± 0.5 years. An age of 18.5 years or older is 2 standard deviations (SD) above the mean, since 17.5 + 1.0 = 18.5 years. The area beyond 2 SD from the mean, on one side of the distribution, represents half of 5%, or 2.5%, which equals 0.025.

10. A research intern in the cardiology department is tasked with reviewing the blood glucose levels of all patients admitted with hypertension-related complications over the past six months. Preliminary data analysis indicates there were 400 such patients, with blood glucose levels following a normal distribution, a mean of 150 mg/dL, and a standard deviation of 15 mg/dL. Given these findings, how many patients in this study are expected to have blood glucose levels ≥180 mg/dL?

A. 5

B. 10

C. 12

D. 20

E. 380

Answer: B. 10. A value of ≥180 mg/dL corresponds to ≥ (150 + 30), or ≥ the mean + 2 standard deviations (SD), which represents 2.5% (0.025) of the population. Since 2.5% of the sample population (400 patients) is 10, the correct answer is 10.

11. A researcher is examining vitamin D levels in a population of elderly individuals living in a region with high rates of osteoporosis. She randomly samples a large group of seniors aged 65 and older and measures their serum vitamin D levels. The results indicate that the data are normally distributed, with a reported mean and standard deviation (SD) for the sample. To account for variability in her sample, she decides to calculate a 95% confidence interval to estimate the average vitamin D level in the entire elderly population. The researcher concludes that the true population mean is likely between 25 and 35 ng/mL. Which calculation was most likely used to derive this confidence interval for the population mean?

    A. Mean ± (SD/√n)

    B. Mean ± 1.96 × (SD/√n)

    C. Mean ± 1.96 × SD

    D. Mean ± 2.58 × (SD/√n)

    E. Mean ± 2.58 × SD

Answer: B. Mean ± 1.96 × (SD/√n). Since the question is about the 95% confidence interval (CI) for the sample mean, we need to use the standard error (SE) instead of the standard deviation (SD). The SE is calculated by dividing the SD by the square root of the sample size (n). While 95% of the distribution is often approximated using a z-score of 2, the exact value for 95% of observations lies within a z-score of 1.96. Therefore, the correct answer is B.

PROBABILITY

This chapter will revise the basic principle of probability and some genetic aspect of probability.

> **LEARNING OUTCOME:**
>
> 1. Define basic probability concepts, such as sample space, independent events, mutually exclusive events and conditional probability.
> 2. Compute probability of specified events (using addition rule and multiplication rule).
> 3. List Hardy-Weinberg equilibrium.
> 4. Analyse probability using Hardy-Weinberg equilibrium.

Probability is the likelihood of an event occurring, expressed as a number between 0 and 1. Each trial in a probability experiment result in an outcome, and the complete set of all possible outcomes is called the sample space. The total probability of all outcomes within the sample space equals 1.

2.1 PROBABILITY RULES FOR MULTIPLE EVENTS

When calculating probabilities, two key rules are applied.

2.1.1 Addition Rule (OR)

A) **Mutually Exclusive Events**: Events A and B cannot occur at the same time (no overlap in outcomes).

Example of mutually exclusive events

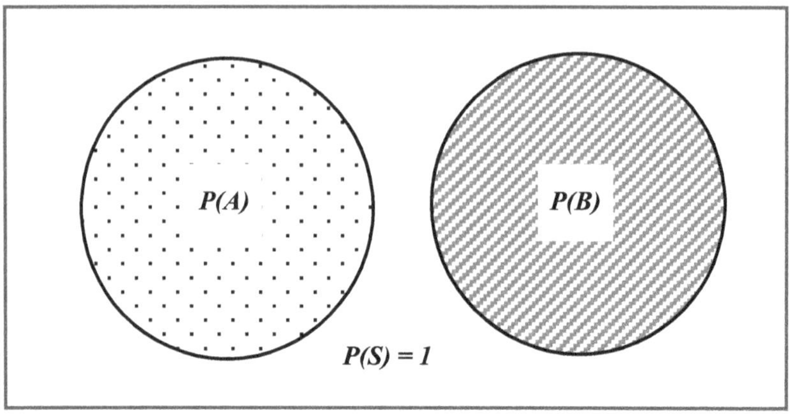

The probability that either A or B occurs is:

P (A OR B) = P(A) + P(B)

B) **Non-mutually Exclusive Events**: Events A and B can occur simultaneously.

Example of non-mutually exclusive events

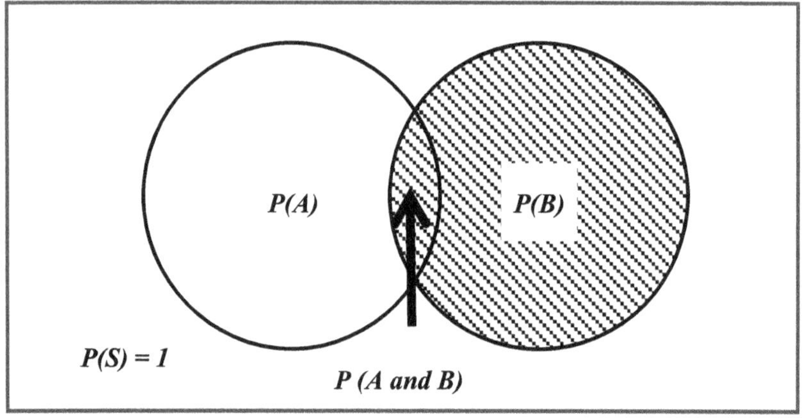

The probability that either A or B occurs is:
P (A OR B) = P(A) + P(B) – P (A AND B)

2.1.2 Multiplication Rule (AND)

A) **Independent Events**: Events A and B are independent if the occurrence of A does not affect the probability of B occurring. For example, the probability of flipping a head on a coin and rolling a 4 on a die.

The probability that both A and B occur is:
$$P (A \text{ AND } B) = P(A) \times P(B)$$

B) **Dependent Events**: Events A and B are dependent if the occurrence of A affects the probability of B occurring.

The probability that both A and B occur, given that A has occurred, is:
$$P(A \text{ AND } B) = P(A) \times P(B \mid A)$$
Conditional Probability ($P(B \mid A)$): The probability that event B occurs given that event A has already occurred is:

$$P (B \mid A) = \frac{P(A \text{ AND } B)}{P(A)}$$

2.2 PROBABILITIES IN GENETICS

2.2.1 Hardy-Weinberg Principle

The Hardy-Weinberg principle is a principle in genetics that describes a state where allele and genotype frequencies in a population will remain stable across generations if no evolutionary forces act on the population.

For a population to achieve Hardy-Weinberg equilibrium, the following conditions must be met:

A) **Large Population Size**: A large population reduces the impact of genetic drift, which causes random changes in allele frequencies. Ideally, the population should be infinitely large.

B) **Random Mating:** All individuals have an equal chance of mating with each other, regardless of their phenotype.

C) **No Natural Selection:** All individuals have an equal chance of surviving and reproducing, with no phenotype offering a survival advantage.

D) **No Migration:** No new individuals with different alleles enter or leave the population.

E) **No Spontaneous Mutations:** There are no new mutations introducing new alleles into the population.

When these conditions are met, the allele frequencies in the population will stay the same, and the genetic variation will remain stable over time. If the frequencies change, it suggests that one or more of these conditions are not being met, indicating that evolutionary forces are at play.

2.2.2 Hardy-Weinberg Analysis

The three types of analysis in Hardy-Weinberg analysis include:

A) **Allele Frequency**: The sum of the frequencies of the normal allele (p) and the mutant allele (q) equals 1:

$$p + q = 1$$

B) **Phenotypic Frequency:** The sum of the frequencies of normal individuals (p^2), carriers (2pq), and diseased individuals (q^2) equals 1:

$$p^2 + 2pq + q^2 = 1$$

C) **Calculating Mutant Allele Frequency from Disease Prevalence:** The frequency of the mutant allele (q) can be determined by taking the square root of the disease prevalence (q^2):

$$q = \sqrt{q^2}$$

▼ **Table 2.1:** Hardy-Weinberg Analysis

Hardy-Weinberg Analysis	
Allele Frequency	p (normal allele frequency) $+$ q (mutant allele frequency) $=$ 1 (Total)
Phenotypic Frequency	p^2 (Frequency of normal individuals) $+$ $2pq$ (Carrier frequency) $+$ q^2 (Frequency of diseased individuals) $=$ 1 (Total)
Calculating Mutant Allele Frequency from Disease Prevalence	q (diseased prevalence) $=$ $\sqrt{q^2}$ (Mutant alleles frequency)

POSSIBLE QUESTIONS FROM THIS CHAPTER

- Calculate the probability using addition rules and multiplication rules
- Identify the conditions required for Hardy-Weinberg equilibrium
- Calculate the alleles frequency
- Calculate the genetic probability using Hardy-Weinberg analysis

Questions on probabilities using addition rules and multiplication rules

12. A pharmaceutical company introduces a novel blood test to screen for a rare liver disease. The test is validated against a liver biopsy, the current gold standard, and shows that it correctly identifies 98% of people without the disease as negative. If this test is used on 10 individuals known to be free of liver disease, what is the likelihood that all 10 results will be negative?

    A. 0.02×10

    B. 0.02^{10}

    C. 0.98×10

    D. 0.98^{10}

    E. $1 - 0.02^{10}$

    F. $1 - 0.98^{10}$

    Answer: D. 0.98^{10}. The probability of a negative result for each individual is 0.98. To find the probability that all 10 individuals are free from liver disease, we apply the multiplication rule.

13. A team of epidemiologists is studying the prevalence of type 2 diabetes among elderly residents of a rural community. The estimated prevalence rates (cases per 100 individuals) based on different age and gender groups are as follows:

Age Group	Women	Men
60-69	15.0	14.5
70-79	20.0	18.0
80-89	25.0	22.0
90+	30.0	28.0
Total	22.0	20.5

During a morning health screening, a physician examines a 62-year-old woman, a 75-year-old man, and an 85-year-old woman from this community. What is the probability that none of them has type 2 diabetes, assuming their conditions are independent of each other?

A. 0.006

B. 0.464

C. 0.553

D. 0.725

E. 0.890

Answer: C. 0.553. As their condition are independent to each other, and none of them to have diabetes, we have to use multiplication rule.

$$= \frac{100-15}{100} \times \frac{100-18}{100} \times \frac{100-25}{100} = 0.85 \times 0.82 \times 0.75 = 0.553$$

Questions on genetic probablities

14. A group of marine biologists is studying the distribution of shell color alleles in a population of sea snails along a coastal region. In a sample of 100 snails, the observed genotype distribution for shell color is as follows: 40 BB (dark shell), 40 Bb (intermediate shell), and 20 bb (light shell). The shell color does not provide any adaptive advantage or disadvantage to the snails in their environment. The population is large and the snails mate randomly. Given this information, is the sea snail population in Hardy-Weinberg equilibrium for the shell color gene?

    A. No, because shell color does not influence survival.

    B. No, because there is an unequal distribution of genotypes.

    C. No, because a higher sample size is needed to confirm equilibrium.

    D. Yes, because random mating and no selection pressure allow for equilibrium.

    Answer: D. Yes, because random mating and no selection pressure allow for equilibrium. The population is large, and the snails mate randomly, which are key conditions for Hardy-Weinberg equilibrium. In addition, the shell color does not provide any adaptive advantage or disadvantage, meaning there is no selection pressure affecting the frequencies of the alleles.

15. A 28-year-old woman and her partner are planning to start a family. She has a family history of cystic fibrosis, and genetic screening reveals that she is a carrier of the Cystic fibrosis transmembrane conductance regulator (CFTR) gene mutation associated with cystic fibrosis, an autosomal recessive condition that affects 1 in 3,600 individuals in the general population. Her partner has no known family history of the disease, and his carrier status is also unknown. What is the probability that their child will be affected by cystic fibrosis?

A. 1/30

B. 1/36

C. 1/60

D. 1/120

E. 1/3,600

F. 1/14,400

Answer: D. 1/120. To determine the probability that the child will inherit the disease, we apply the multiplication rule by combining three probabilities: the probability of the mother passing the mutation to the child (which is ½, as the mother is a carrier), the probability of the father passing the mutation (which is ½ if the father is a carrier), and the probability that the father is a carrier. The probability of the partner being a carrier is calculated as follows: Cystic fibrosis is an autosomal recessive disorder, and 1 in 3,600 individuals in the general population are affected. This means that the frequency of affected individuals (q^2) is $\dfrac{1}{3600}$. Using Hardy-Weinberg equilibrium, the carrier frequency ($2pq$) is estimated: $q^2 = \dfrac{1}{3600}, q = \dfrac{1}{\sqrt{3600}} = \dfrac{1}{60}$. If $q = \dfrac{1}{60}$, then the carrier frequency $2pq$ is approximately:

$$2pq \approx 2 \times \frac{1}{59} \times \frac{1}{60} \approx \frac{1}{30}.$$ Thus, there is a 1/30 chance that her partner is a carrier of the CFTR mutation.

The total probability that the child will inherit the mutation from both parents is: $\text{Total probability} = \dfrac{1}{30} \times \dfrac{1}{2} \times \dfrac{1}{2} = \dfrac{1}{120}$

16. A team of geneticists is studying a particular gene in a species of frogs that exhibits two allelic variants, B and D. Frogs with BB and BD genotypes show the dominant phenotype, while frogs with DD genotype express the recessive trait. In a population of 500 frogs, the following genotype distribution is observed:

Genotype	Number of Frogs
BB	200
BD	220
DD	80

Which of the following represents the frequency of the D allele in the frog population?

A. 80/500

B. 220/500

C. 160/1000

D. 300/1000

E. 380/1000

F. 440/1000

Answer: E. 380/1000.

$$Frequency\ of\ D\ alleles = \frac{D\ alleles}{total\ alleles} = \frac{homozygous\ recessive\ frogs\,(2) + heterozygous\ frogs}{number\ of\ frogs\,(2)} = \frac{(80 \times 2) + 220}{500 \times 2} = \frac{380}{1000}$$

MEASURE OF DISEASE FREQUENCY

This chapter introduces the most common epidemiological measures used to assess disease frequency, shedding light on the tools and techniques that quantify how often diseases arise and spread across various groups.

LEARNING OUTCOME:

1. Calculate incidence, prevalence, attack rate and case fatality rate.
2. Compare and contrast incidence and prevalence and factors affecting them.
3. Identify application of incidence and prevalence.
4. List characteristics of different types of population pyramid and differentiate them.

Epidemiology examines the patterns and causes of diseases in populations. A key part of this field involves understanding how disease frequency is measured, which is essential for identifying trends in disease distribution.

3.1 COMMON MEASURE OF DISEASE FREQUENCY

The two most crucial and widely used measures in epidemiology are prevalence and incidence.

3.1.1 Incidence

Incidence of a disease is the number of new cases that develop in a population at risk for the diseases over a specific period of time.

A) Cumulative incidence (Attack Rate)

It is the proportion of people in a pre-defined group of fixed size (fixed cohort) who develop the disease during a specified time period. This assumes that all individuals in the at-risk population are followed up either until they develop the disease or until the observation period concludes.

It can be used to assess the risk (probability) that a healthy individual will develop the disease in question during a specified period.

Calculation

$$cumulative\,incidence = \frac{\text{number of new cases during the specified time period}}{\text{total number of people at risk}}$$

NB:

Numerator – only new cases (ongoing cases are exclude)

Denominator – existing cases are excluded (if the diseases is incurable)

B) Incidence density (incidence rate, hazard rate, and force of morbidity or mortality)

It refers to the rate at which new cases or deaths occur within a population, accounting for the fact that individuals are observed for varying lengths of time and are at risk throughout the study period. Variations in the number of individuals studied and the duration of observation are a result of real-world study conditions.

Incidence density measures the average rate at which a disease develops in a population over a defined period.

Calculation

$$incidence\,density = \frac{\text{number of new cases of disease during specified time period}}{\text{person} - \text{time at risk for disease}}$$

3.1.2 Prevalence

Prevalence of a disease in a population is the proportion of that population having the disorder at a given point in time.

Calculation

$$prevalence = \frac{\text{Total number of diseased individuals at given time}}{\text{total population}}$$

NB:

Numerator – both new and ongoing cases of the disease

Example

Cases of xx [= onset of disease

——] = duration of diseases

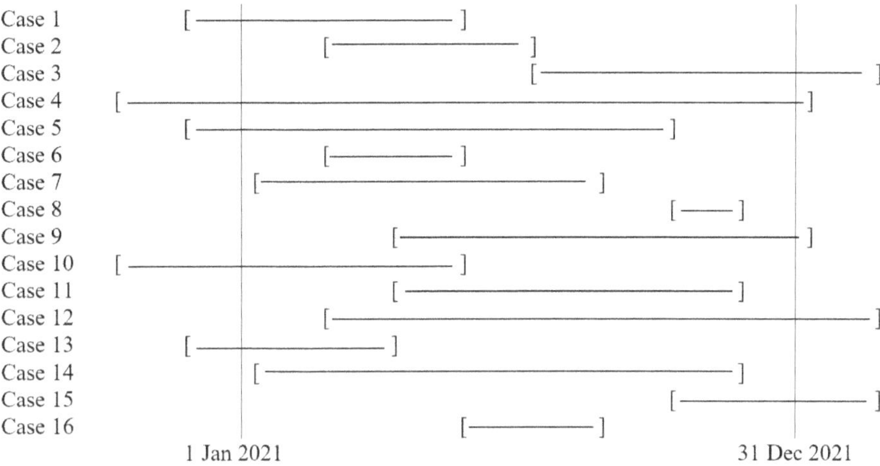

1 January 2021, 5 out of 16 have disease X

Prevalence of disease X on 1 January 2021 is 5/16

3.1.3 Case Fatality

Case fatality rate is an indicator of disease severity. It measures the proportion of individuals diagnosed with a particular disease who die from it.

$$case\ fatality\,(\%) = \frac{\text{No. of people dying during a specified period of time after the disease diagnosis}}{\text{No. of individuals with that specified diagnos}} \times 100\%$$

3.1.4 Factors Affecting the Incidence and Prevalence

Prevalence decreases with

decrease incidence, increased mortality, shorter duration of disease, improved treatment

Incidence decreases with

Improved resistance to disease and effective intervention program

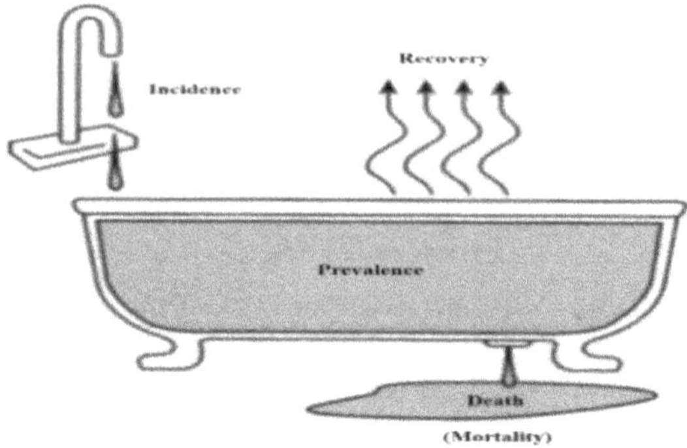

▲ **Figure 3.1:** Factors affecting on incidence and prevalence

3.1.5 Practical Application

The practical applications of incidence and prevalence in public health and epidemiology are distinct but complementary.

A) Incidence:

1. **Assessing Disease Risk:** Incidence measures the rate at which new cases of a disease occur in a population over a specific period. It helps identify populations at higher risk of developing a disease.

   Example: Incidence data can track how fast a new infectious disease, like COVID-19, is spreading within a community.

2. **Evaluating Intervention Effectiveness:** By comparing incidence rates before and after a public health intervention (e.g., vaccination campaigns or preventive measures), the success of the intervention can be assessed.

   Example: Decreases in the incidence of cervical cancer after the introduction of the HPV vaccine.

3. **Outbreak Monitoring and Response:** Incidence is used to detect and respond to disease outbreaks in real-time, guiding urgent public health measures.

   Example: Monitoring weekly incidence rates of seasonal influenza to determine when flu outbreaks are intensifying.

B) Prevalence:

1. **Estimating Disease Burden:** Prevalence measures the total number of existing cases (both new and old) at a specific point in time or over a period, reflecting the overall disease burden on a population.

   Example: Estimating the number of people living with diabetes in a country to plan healthcare resources.

2. **Healthcare Resource Allocation:** Prevalence data informs healthcare planners on the demand for treatment, services, and long-term care facilities, especially for chronic diseases.

   Example: High prevalence of heart disease might lead to an increased need for cardiologists, rehabilitation centres, and medications.

3. **Identifying Public Health Priorities:** High-prevalence conditions often become public health priorities because they require sustained resources and policy attention.

   Example: The prevalence of mental health disorders may guide mental health programs and support services.

Together, incidence helps in understanding the spread and control of diseases, while prevalence provides insight into the overall disease burden and the long-term needs of a population.

3.2 POPULATION PYRAMID

A population pyramid is a graphical representation that illustrates the age and sex distribution of a population, whether of a country or a region. Population pyramids are generally categorized into three types: stationary, expansive, or constrictive, based on a country's fertility and mortality rates.

3.2.1 Expansive Pyramid

An expansive or expanding population pyramid is typical of countries with high birth rates and low life expectancy (high death rates). These populations are fast-growing, with each birth cohort increasing in size, resulting in a broad base representing the younger age groups.

3.2.2 Stationary Pyramid

A stationary or constant population pyramid occurs when birth and death rates are roughly balanced. In this scenario, the proportions of the population across age and sex groups remain relatively stable over time.

3.2.3 Constrictive Pyramid

A constrictive or declining population pyramid is characteristic of highly developed countries with high levels of education, access to birth control, good healthcare, and longer life expectancy. These populations experience low birth and death rates, leading to an older average age and a high dependency ratio due to fewer people of working age. The base of the pyramid is narrower, reflecting the smaller younger population.

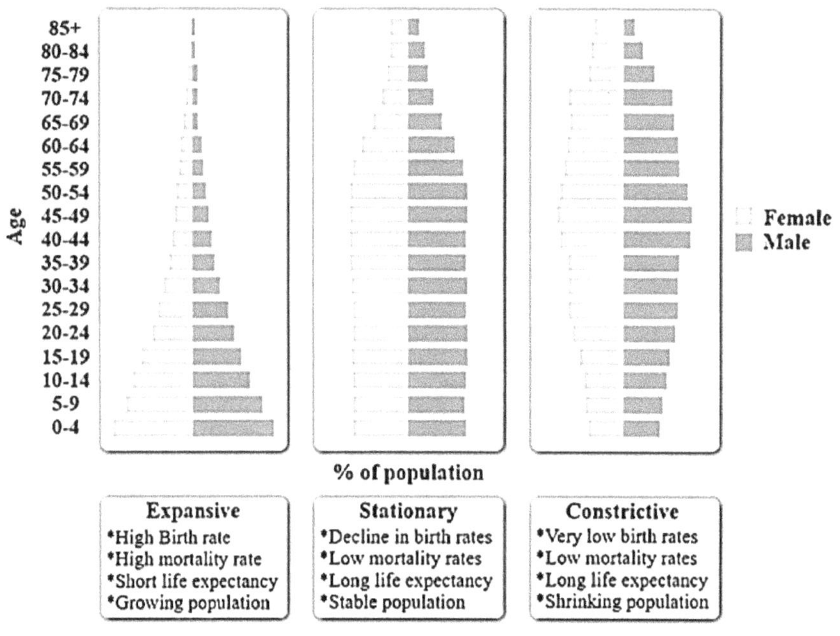

▲ **Figure 3.2:** Different Types of Population Pyramid

Possible question from this chapter

- Calculate the Incidence, Prevalence, Attack rate, Case Fatality Rate
- Identify the factors influencing the incidence and prevalence
- Identify the characteristics of the population from population pyramid

Questions on calculation of Incidence, Prevalence, attack rate and case fatality rate

17. A public health team is conducting a study to assess the prevalence of ventilator-associated pneumonia (VAP) in the intensive care unit (ICU) of a large teaching hospital. The graph below displays the number of active VAP cases reported each day in the ICU during the month of October. Based on the data presented, what is the number of prevalent cases on October 31?

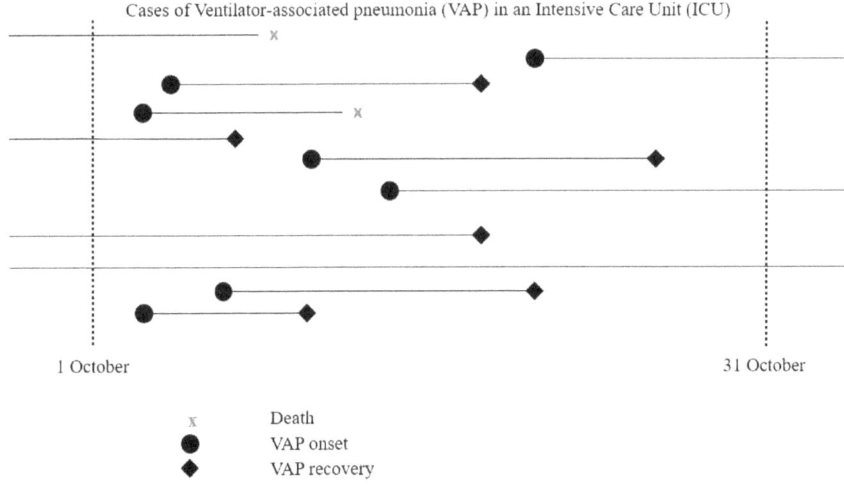

A. 3

B. 4

C. 6

D. 7

E. 11

Answer: A.3. The total number of people with VAP on 31 October is 3.

18. In 2018, a state with a population of 3,500,000 recorded 20,000 cases of a specific viral infection at the start of the year. By the end of the same year, an additional 5,000 cases were diagnosed, and 800 people had died from the infection. The state also recorded 30,000 deaths from other unrelated causes. What was the cumulative incidence of the infection in 2018?

    A. 800 / 30,000

    B. 800/3,500,000

    C. 5,000/ 3,500,000

    D. 25,000/3,500,000

    E. 5,000/3,480,000

    F. 25,000/3,480,000

    G. 5,000/3,450,000

    Answer: E. 5000/3,480,000. The numerator is new cases which is 5,000 and the denominator is the number of people who are at risk which is $3,480,000 \ (3,500,000 - 20,000)$.

19. A local community centre held a holiday party where a buffet meal was served. The menu included turkey, stuffing, and green beans. The following day, 35 out of the 120 attendees reported nausea and vomiting. Attendees were surveyed about the foods they had eaten, and the following table was obtained:

Food item or combination of items	Number of attendees who ate food item or combination of items	Number of attendees who developed nausea and vomiting
Turkey only	25	4
Stuffing only	20	3
Green beans only	15	1
Turkey and stuffing	30	9
Turkey and green beans	10	3
Stuffing and green beans	10	5
Turkey, stuffing, and green beans	10	4

Which of the following best describes the attack rate among all attendees who had stuffing?

A. 10%

B. 12%

C. 14%

D. 18%

E. 22%

F. 26%

G. 30%

Answer: G. 30%.

$$\text{attack rate} = \frac{\text{eat stuffings and develop symptoms}}{\text{all stuffing eaters}} = \frac{3+9+5+4}{20+30+10+10} = \frac{30}{100} = 30\%$$

20. A regional hospital is conducting an annual review of its infectious disease control program. The infection rates and outcomes for community-acquired pneumonia in the hospital's emergency department are summarized in the table below for the last year:

Infection Type	Number of Fatal Cases	% of All Fatal Cases	Number of Nonfatal Cases	% of All Nonfatal Cases
S. pneumoniae	12	15	50	20
K. pneumoniae	30	37	100	40
H. influenzae	20	25	60	25
Viral pneumonia	10	12	30	12
Other	9	11	10	3
Total	81	100	250	100

What is the case-fatality rate for *K. pneumoniae* pneumonia in this hospital?

A. 30/81

B. 30/100

C. 30/130

D. 30/250

E. 100/250

Answer: C. 30/130. The total number of cases of *Klebsiella pneumoniae* pneumonia is 130 (30 fatal + 100 non-fatal). Among these, 30 cases resulted in death. Therefore, the case fatality rate for *Klebsiella pneumoniae* pneumonia is 30 out of 130.

Questions on factors affection incidence and prevalence

21. A chronic lung disease has been prevalent among a specific population of coal miners. Over the past few years, due to government policies, the number of healthy miners left the profession. No changes have occurred in the treatment or prevention of the disease. What is the most likely effect of this on the prevalence of the disease among the mining population?

    A. The prevalence would decrease

    B. The prevalence would increase

    C. The prevalence would remain the same

    D. It is not possible to determine the effect on prevalence from the information given.

    Answer: B. The prevalence would increase. As healthy individuals leave the profession, the denominator decreases, while the numerator remains unchanged, since those leaving are healthy. This results in a higher proportion of individuals with the disease within the remaining population.

22. An epidemiological study has been launched to evaluate the impact of systemic lupus erythematosus in a large, stable population with minimal migration. The incidence and prevalence of the disease are tracked and documented as the number of cases per 100,000 people over an 8-year span.

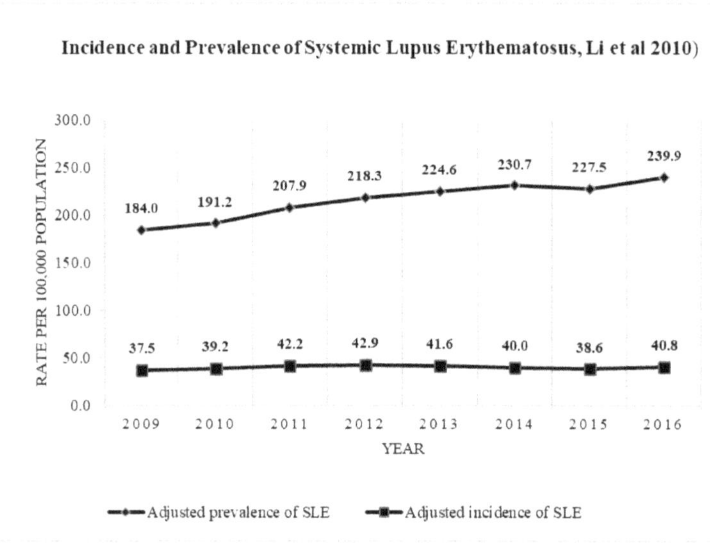

Incidence and Prevalence of Systemic Lupus Erythematosus, Li et al 2010)

Which of the following is the most likely explanation for the change in disease prevalence seen in the graph?

A. Decreased hospitalization rate

B. Improved quality of care

C. Increased exposure to risk factors

D. Increased mortality in SLE

E. Increased number of new SLE cases

F. Increased precision of diagnostic testing

G. Selective survival bias

Answer: B. Improved quality of care. Regardless of a similar incidence rate, an increase in prevalence typically indicates that patients are living longer due to lower mortality, most likely as a result of improved quality of care.

23. A 58-year-old woman is diagnosed with advanced ovarian cancer. A new drug, designed to target cancerous cells without harming healthy tissues, has been introduced. Clinical trials show that this drug significantly extends survival in patients with advanced ovarian cancer but does not provide a cure. If this drug becomes widely available, what changes would be expected in the number of incident and prevalent cases of ovarian cancer?

    A. The number of incident cases will decrease, the number of prevalent cases will decrease

    B. The number of incident cases will decrease, the number of prevalent cases will increase

    C. The number of incident cases will increase, the number of prevalent cases will not change

    D. The number of incident cases will not change, the number of prevalent cases will increase

    E. The number of incident cases will not change, the number of prevalent cases will not change

Answer: D. The number of incident cases will not change, the number of prevalent cases will increase. Since this drug significantly extends survival in patients with advanced ovarian cancer without providing a cure, it would not affect the incidence of the disease. However, it would increase the prevalence, as the number of patients would rise due to longer survival.

Questions on characteristics of population based on population pyramid

24. The population pyramid of Italy is seen as below.

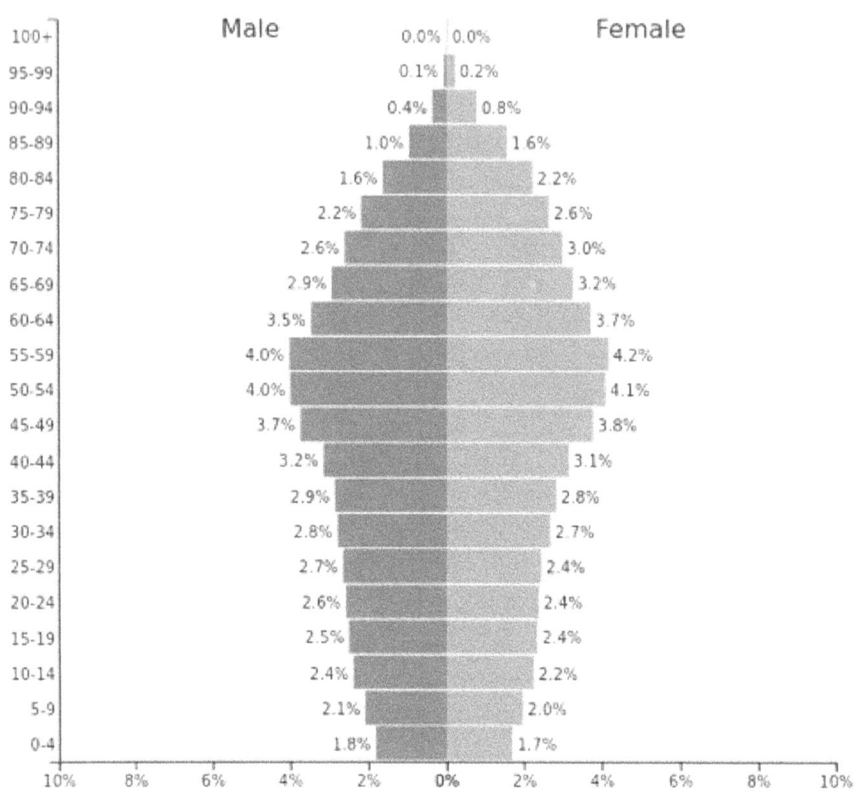

Based on the population pyramid, which of the following is most likely true about Italy and its population?

A. Italy seems to have a high birth rate; therefore, the population must be growing.

B. Italy seems to have a high death rate; therefore, the population must be shrinking.

C. Italy seems to have a low birth rate; therefore, the population must be old.

D. Italy seems to have a short life expectancy; therefore, the population must be young.

E. Italy seems to have a similar percentage of people in each age cohort; therefore, the population must be stable.

Answer: C. Italy seems to have a low birth rate; therefore, the population must be old. The population consists of a larger proportion of older people compared to younger ones.

EPIDEMIOLOGICAL METHODS

This chapter will introduce commonly used epidemiological study design.

LEARNING OUTCOME:

1. Identify the epidemiological study design based on the scenario.
2. Select the appropriate samples.
3. Differentiate different phases of clinical trials.

4.1 BROAD CLASSIFICATION OF EPIDEMIOLOGICAL STUDIES

Research can be broadly classified into qualitative and quantitative designs. **Qualitative research studies** employ methods like focus groups, structured and semi-structured interviews, and other anthropological techniques to gather narrative data that offer deeper insights and better understanding of trends or patterns in quantitative findings. On the other hand, **quantitative research studies** are systematic and structured approach to studying phenomena. It involves collecting measurable data and applying statistical, mathematical, or computational techniques for analysis.

Quantitative studies are typically categorized into observational or experimental designs, depending on the level of control the researcher has over the independent variables (e.g., exposure to risk factors, treatments). The primary differences between these two study designs are as follows:

A) **observational designs**: The researcher passively observes the outcomes related to naturally occurring risk factors or exposures, without intervening as in experimental studies. Here, the researcher has no control over the independent variables (e.g., exposure to risk factors, treatments). Case series, cross-sectional studies, case-control studies, cohort studies (both retrospective and prospective), and hybrid designs are observational studies

B) **experimental designs**: The researcher actively controls and usually randomly assigns interventions to participants to assess their effects. This allows for controlled manipulation of the independent variables (e.g., treatments, interventions, exposure to risk factors).

4.2 OBSERVATIONAL STUDIES

Observational studies can be further divided into:

A) **Descriptive studies**, which collect data to characterize specific health problems (e.g., disease prevalence, incidence rates).

B) **Analytical studies**, which test hypotheses to evaluate the associations between risk factors and disease.

4.2.1 Case Series Study

A case series is a descriptive observational study design that focuses on a typically small group of patients with a similar diagnosis or treatment, observed at a specific point in time or over a certain period. It tracks patients with a known condition (such as exposure, risk factor, or disease) to document their natural history or response to treatment. Unlike other observational designs, such as cohort or case-control studies, a case series is purely descriptive, lacks a comparison group, and cannot establish associations between risk factors (such as treatment or exposure) and outcomes (such as diseases or complications), nor can it quantify statistical significance.

4.2.2 Cross-Sectional Study

A cross-sectional study is an observational study that assesses a population of interest at a single point in time, commonly used to estimate disease prevalence and its association with specific risk factors. Also known as a prevalence study, it involves the simultaneous measurement of both exposure and outcome, providing a snapshot of the population. This study design is frequently employed in surveys because it is relatively inexpensive and easy to conduct. In a cross-sectional study, individuals are randomly selected from the population based on predefined inclusion and exclusion criteria, and their exposure status and outcomes are simultaneously determined. For instance, participants might be randomly selected from a region with high tuberculosis prevalence and categorized based on a risk factor (e.g., vaping) and an outcome (e.g., tuberculosis status). The primary aim is to determine prevalence by capturing a snapshot of the population.

Unlike other observational designs, such as cohort or case-control studies, cross-sectional studies do not establish a clear temporal relationship between exposure and outcome (i.e., they do not separate the time period of exposure from the outcome). This lack of temporal distinction is a significant limitation, as it hinders the ability to draw causal conclusions. While cross-sectional studies can evaluate associations between risk factors and outcomes, they cannot establish causality.

4.2.3 Case-Control Study

A case-control study is an analytical observational design that involves selecting two groups of individuals: those who have the outcome of interest (cases) and those who do not (controls). The selection of cases and controls is based on disease status, not exposure status. Controls are chosen to provide an accurate estimation of exposure frequency in the non-diseased general population.

Once the groups are selected, the frequency of exposure to specific risk factors (e.g., chemical waste, lead) is determined for both cases and controls. The exposure frequency is then compared between the two groups to estimate the association between the risk factors and the outcomes. If a statistically significant difference in exposure frequency is found between the groups, it suggests that the risk factor may be associated with the development of the disease. This study design is particularly suited for evaluating rare conditions.

For example, to investigate the association between lead exposure and cognitive deficits, a case-control study might be conducted. Children with cognitive deficits would be selected as cases, while those without cognitive deficits would serve as controls. After identifying the cases and controls, researchers would retrospectively assess exposure to the risk factor of interest, such as lead exposure. The association would be determined by comparing the frequency of lead exposure among cases and controls.

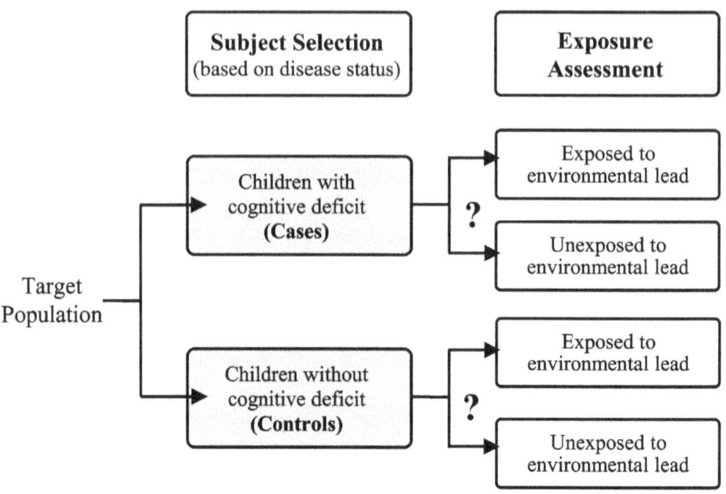

▲ **Figure 4.1. Case Control study design**

4.2.4 Cohort Study

A cohort study is an observational analytic study design where the term "cohort" refers to a group of individuals sharing similar characteristics, often with the same exposure status. In a cohort study, participants are initially selected from a population of interest. Once categorized based on their exposure status to a particular risk factor, they are followed over time to assess the occurrence (i.e., incidence) of the outcome of interest in each group during the study period. The occurrence of the outcome is then compared between the exposed and non-exposed groups to estimate the association between the risk factors and the outcomes. This design is particularly well-suited for evaluating rare exposures.

For instance, to investigate the association between lead exposure and cognitive deficits using a cohort study, two groups of individuals (cohorts) would be identified based on their environmental lead exposure status. These groups would be followed over time to determine the incidence of cognitive deficits. The association is then calculated by comparing the incidence of cognitive deficits between individuals exposed to lead and those who were not.

There are two types of cohort studies: prospective cohort and retrospective cohort studies.

- In prospective cohort studies, the exposure status is determined in the present, and participants are tracked over time for the development of the outcome of interest.

- In retrospective cohort studies, the exposure status is determined at a specific point in the past, and participants are followed retrospectively, typically through medical records.

Sometimes, even if the exposure status is determined retrospectively using medical records, the outcome is yet known and patients are tracked from the point of exposure onward, it is still considered a prospective cohort study.

Unlike experimental studies, participants in cohort studies already have a defined exposure status; they are not randomly assigned to exposed or non-exposed groups.

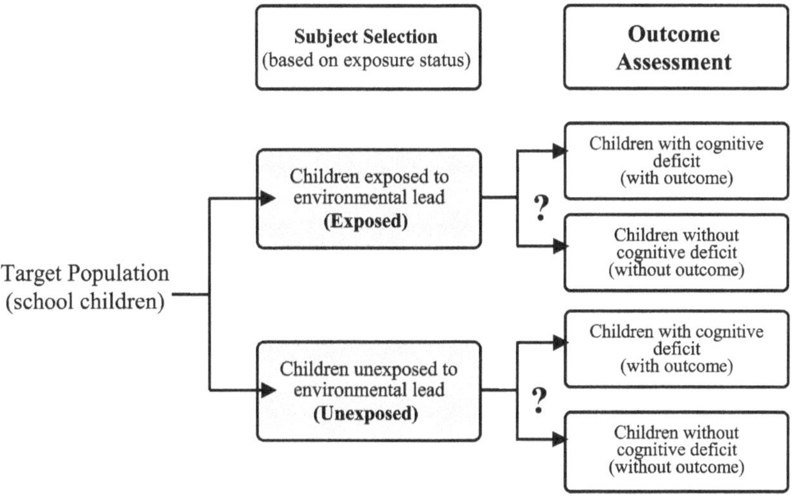

▲ Figure 4.2. Cohort study design

4.2.5 Hybrid Designs

The most common hybrid designs are nested case-control studies and nested case-cohort studies. The term "nested" indicates that these studies are embedded within larger cohort studies.

Nested case-control studies begin within the framework of a cohort study, where participants are followed over time. Those who develop the outcome of interest become the cases for the case-control study, while controls are selected from cohort members who have not developed the disease during the same period. The key advantage of this design is that cases and controls are more comparable than in traditional case-control designs since they come from the same well-defined population, thereby minimizing potential selection bias.

In nested case-cohort studies, a random sample is selected from all members of the cohort at the beginning of the study, rather than selecting controls only from those who do not develop the disease. During the analytic phase, participants who develop the outcomes are identified and analysed.

4.2.6 Ecological Study

An ecological study is an observational study that uses population-level data, rather than individual-level data, as the unit of analysis to evaluate the association between a potential exposure (e.g., low socioeconomic status) and a given outcome (e.g., increased cancer mortality). In some cases, ecological studies may involve multiple countries, relying on population-level data rather than individual-level data. Unlike case-control and cohort studies, which focus on individuals, the unit of analysis in ecological studies is the population as a whole.

Ecological studies are useful for generating hypotheses but should not be used to draw conclusions about individuals within these populations. A significant drawback of this type of study is the risk of encountering an ecological fallacy.

4.3 EXPERIMENTAL STUDIES

Experimental studies are analytical studies designed to test hypotheses about the relationship between specific exposures and outcomes. Unlike observational studies, the investigator has direct control over the study conditions. A clinical trial is a type of experimental study in which patients are prospectively assigned to two or more interventions (often including a placebo or control treatment) to evaluate the effects of those interventions on outcomes of interest.

For example, patients who underwent colostomy surgery were randomly assigned to either an antibiotic-ointment treatment group or a standard-of-care control group. The effectiveness of the antibiotic ointment in preventing surgical-site infections was then assessed by recording the incidence and severity of infections in each group.

4.3.1 Randomized Controlled Trial

A randomized controlled trial (RCT) is a subtype of experimental design in which participants are randomly allocated to two or more groups to assess the effect of specific interventions (e.g., treatments). Typically, subjects are randomly assigned to either a treatment arm or a placebo (control arm) and then followed to observe the development of the outcome of interest.

When groups differ significantly in characteristics such as disease severity, the effect of a treatment may be underestimated or overestimated, depending on which group has a higher proportion of severe cases. Random assignment of subjects to experimental groups helps to balance these variables, ensuring that the groups are as similar as possible, except for the treatment assignment. This process, known as randomization, aims to ensure that any differences observed between the groups are due exclusively to the treatment and not to other underlying factors.

The success of randomization is evaluated by analysing the similarity of underlying variables (e.g., sex, age, weight, disease severity) between the groups, and the results are reported in a baseline characteristics table. Randomization helps prevent selection bias and increases the likelihood that any differences observed between groups are due solely to the treatment rather than to other characteristics.

4.3.2 Crossover Study

A crossover study is an experiment in which subjects are sequentially exposed to different treatments or exposures. Patients are randomly assigned to a sequence of treatment groups. The simplest model is an AB/BA study, where Group A receives the active treatment and Group B receives a placebo. After the initial treatment period, the treatments are switched: Group A receives the placebo, and Group B receives the active treatment. This design allows patients to serve as their own controls.

The main drawback of crossover trials is the potential carryover effect, where the effects of one treatment may influence the response to a subsequent treatment. To mitigate this, a washout phase (a period without treatment) is often included between treatments to allow the effects of the previous treatment to wear off.

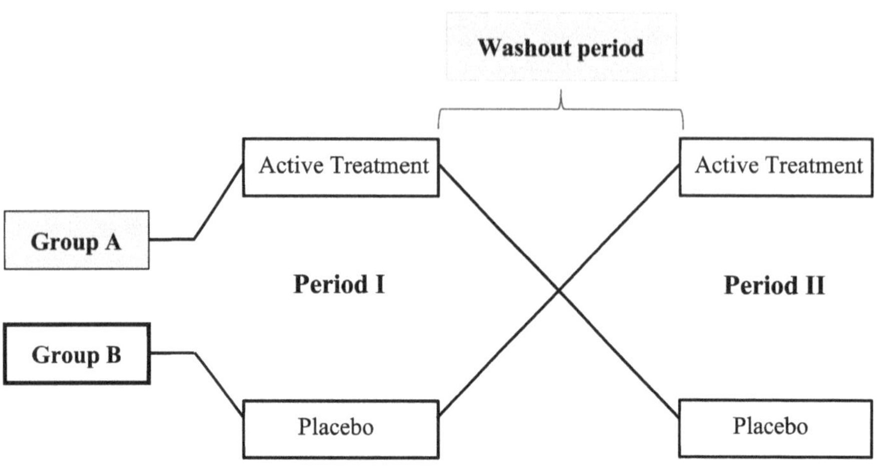

▲ **Figure 4.3:** Cross-over study design

4.3.3 Blinded Studies

A blind study is a type of clinical trial in which either the participants (single-blind), the researchers (single-blind), or both the participants and the researchers (double-blind) are unaware of the treatment assignments. Although randomization is used to assign patients to treatment groups, it does not automatically ensure that the study is blinded.

4.3.4 Phases of Clinical Trials

Clinical trials are divided into a preclinical phase and four clinical phases:

A) **Preclinical Phase (Laboratory Phase):** This phase involves laboratory research using animal models to explore whether and how a new treatment might work.

B) **Clinical Phase I (Human Safety):** In this phase, a small number of healthy volunteers are studied to assess the treatment's safety, toxicity, pharmacokinetics, pharmacodynamics, and the maximum tolerated dose.

C) **Clinical Phase II (Expanded Human Safety):** This phase involves a small group of affected patients to evaluate the treatment's efficacy, determine optimal dosing, and monitor for adverse effects.

D) **Clinical Phase III (Efficacy and Safety Comparison):** A larger group of affected patients is randomly assigned to either the new treatment or the best available standard treatment. This phase compares the new treatment to the current standard of care.

E) **Clinical Phase IV (Post-Marketing Surveillance):** After the treatment is approved, this phase involves monitoring affected patients to identify rare and long-term adverse effects, ensuring ongoing safety and efficacy.

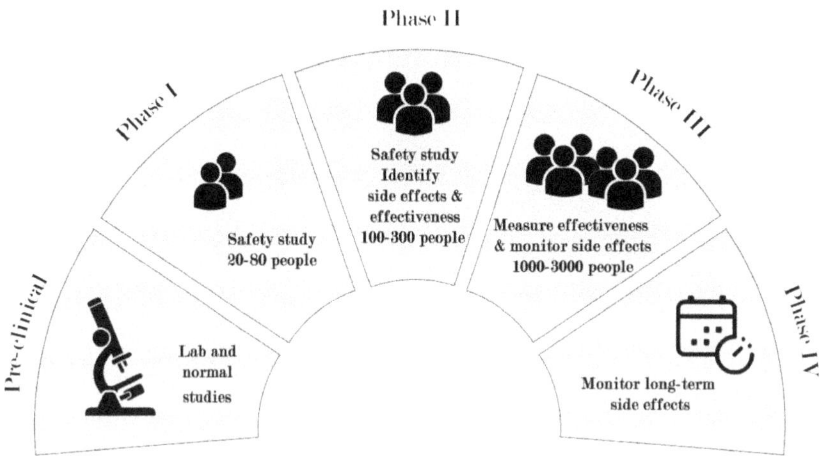

▲ **Figure 4.4:** Phases of clinical trials

4.4   SYSTEMATIC REVIEWS AND META-ANALYSES

Systematic reviews and meta-analyses aggregate the results of multiple published studies, particularly focusing on high-quality randomized controlled trials, to estimate the overall pooled effect aggregate the results of multiple published studies, particularly focusing on high-quality randomized controlled trials, to estimate the overall pooled effect.

4.5 TEMPORALITY OF DIFFERENT STUDY DESIGNS

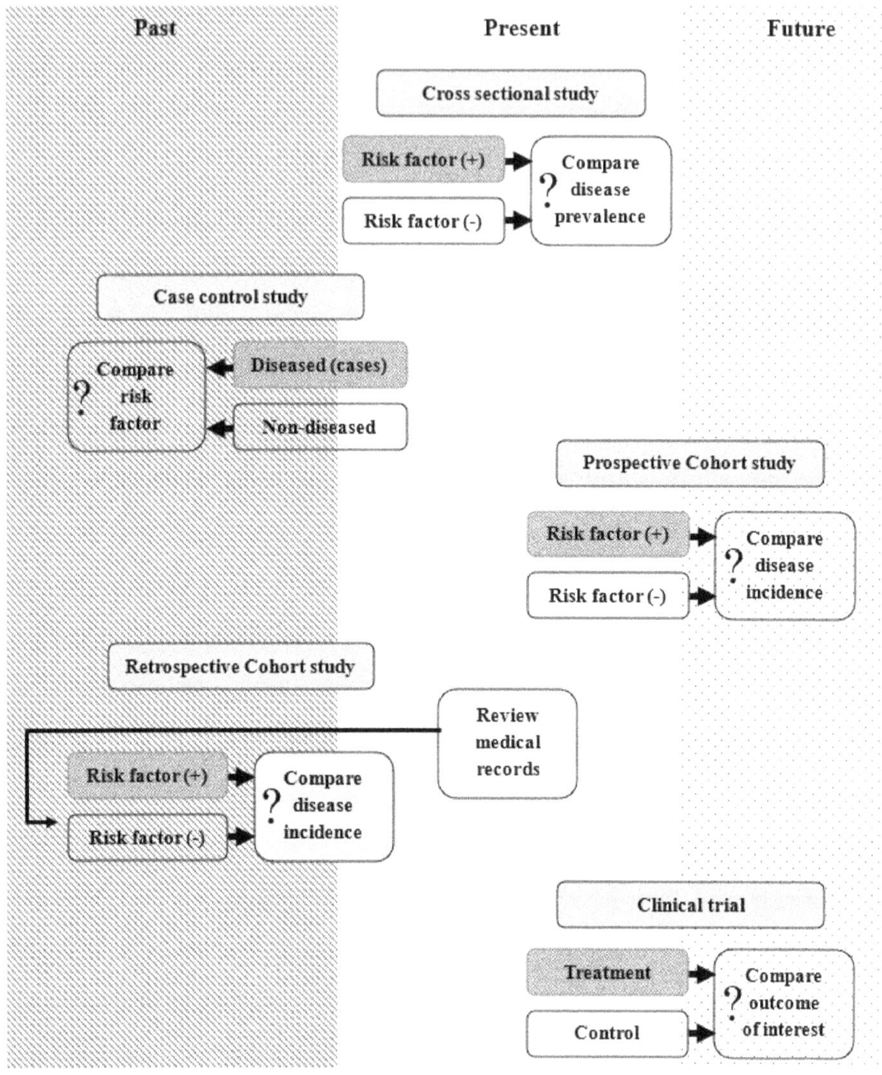

▲ **Figure 4.5:** Temporality of different study designs

4.6 REPORT OF FINDINGS BASED ON STUDY DESIGNS

Due to its retrospective nature, a case-control study cannot compare the frequency (i.e., incidence, risk, rate) of events that occur after a disease has been diagnosed (i.e., prospective outcomes). Prospective outcomes are more appropriately studied in cohort studies and experimental designs.

In case-control studies, the measure of association between a risk factor and an outcome is typically expressed as an odds ratio. This compares the odds of exposure to a particular characteristic (e.g., consumption of specific food) between affected individuals (e.g., patients with cancer) and unaffected individuals who serve as controls.

In cohort studies, the measure of association between a risk factor and an outcome is usually presented as relative risk. This compares the risk of developing an outcome (e.g., cancer) between individuals exposed to a particular characteristic (e.g., consumption of specific food) and those who are not exposed.

Possible questions from this chapter

- Identify the study designs.
- Identify the phases of clinical trials.
- Identify the appropriate measure of interest (risk factors) in case-control study.
- Identify the appropriate comparison group for cohort study.
- Identify the appropriate control for case control study.
- Identify the purpose of randomization.

Questions on identification of study designs

25. A group of doctors is investigating the neurological complications of a new type of viral infection. They collect data from 10 patients who experienced seizures during the course of their illness. The study reports detailed information about the patients' symptoms, diagnostic results, and treatment outcomes, without including a control group or making comparisons. Which of the following best describes this study design?

    A. Case series

    B. Case-control study

    C. Clinical trial

    D. Cohort

    E. Cross-sectional

    Answer: A. Case series. This study presents observations from a small group of patients with similar conditions, making it a case series study.

26. A group of researchers is investigating the association between high cholesterol levels and the prevalence of type 2 diabetes in a population. They randomly select a group of individuals, measure their cholesterol levels, and collect information on whether they currently have type 2 diabetes. The data is collected at a single point in time, and the researchers analyze the relationship between cholesterol levels and diabetes. Which of the following best describes this study design?

A. Case-control study

B. Cross-sectional study

C. Prospective cohort study

D. Randomized clinical trial

E. Retrospective cohort study

Answer: B. Cross-sectional study. Collecting data at a single point in time classifies this as a cross-sectional study.

27. Researchers aim to investigate the potential link between exposure to secondhand smoke and the development of asthma in children. They select 50 children with a diagnosis of asthma from local clinics and match them with 50 children without asthma from the same clinics. The researchers then interview the parents to determine the children's history of exposure to secondhand smoke in the household. Which of the following best describes this study design?

A. Case series study

B. Case-control study

C. Cross-sectional study

D. Prospective cohort study

E. Randomized control trial

Answer: B. Case-control study. The history of secondhand smoke exposure is compared between individuals with asthma (cases) and those without asthma (controls), making this a case-control study.

28. A team of researchers is studying the impact of a high-fat diet on the development of heart disease. In 2005, they selected a group of 5,000 individuals who followed a high-fat diet and another group of 5,000 individuals who followed a low-fat diet. They collected baseline data on diet, exercise, and medical history. These participants were followed over a period of 15 years, with regular check-ups to monitor the incidence of heart disease. What is the MOST appropriate study design for this research?

A. Case-control study

B. Cohort study

C. Cross-sectional study

D. Ecological study

E. Randomized clinical trial

Answer B: Cohort study. In this study, the researcher followed patients over time to observe the occurrence of heart disease based on their dietary fat exposure, making it a cohort study design.

29. In 2020, a researcher wanted to examine the long-term effects of occupational exposure to asbestos. The researcher looked at the medical records of 2,000 factory workers who were employed between 1980 and 2000, dividing them into two groups based on their levels of asbestos exposure. The workers' health data from 2000 to 2020 were analyzed to determine the incidence of lung cancer and other respiratory diseases. Which of the following best describes the study design?

A. Case-control study

B. Cross-sectional study

C. Prospective cohort study

D. Randomized clinical trial

E. Retrospective cohort study

Answer: E. Retrospective cohort study. While the exposure status is assessed retrospectively, participants are classified based on their exposure, and the outcomes are then tracked over time. Therefore, this is not a case-control study; instead, it is a retrospective cohort study.

30. A research team is investigating the relationship between air pollution and the prevalence of asthma across different cities in Europe. The researchers collected data from each city's environmental agencies on air pollution levels over the last decade, as well as citywide asthma hospitalization rates reported by local health departments. The data were analyzed to determine if cities with higher pollution levels had higher asthma rates. Which of the following best describes the design of this study?

    A. Case-control study

    B. Cohort study

    C. Cross-sectional survey

    D. Ecological study

    E. Randomized controlled trial

    Answer D: Ecological study. The unit of analysis in this study is at the population level, comparing the prevalence of asthma with air pollution levels across different cities. Therefore, this is classified as an ecological study.

31. Researchers are studying whether a specific type of diet can help patients with Type 2 diabetes control their blood sugar levels. One hundred patients with Type 2 diabetes are randomly assigned to either a low-carbohydrate diet or a standard diabetic diet. Both groups follow their assigned diets for 12 months, and their blood sugar levels are monitored monthly. At the end of the study, the groups' blood sugar control is compared to see which diet was more effective. Which of the following best describes the study design?

    A. Case-control study

    B. Crossover design

    C. Cross-sectional study

    D. Prospective cohort study

    E. Randomized controlled trial

    Answer E: Randomized Controlled Trial. In this study, the researcher randomly assigned patients to either a low-carbohydrate diet or a standard diabetic diet, making it a randomized controlled trial.

32. A study is conducted to compare the effects of two different sleep aids, melatonin and daridorexant, on sleep quality in adults with insomnia. Thirty participants are randomly assigned to two groups. One group receives melatonin for two weeks, while the other group receives a daridorexant. After a one-week washout period, the groups switch treatments for another two weeks. Sleep quality is measured using a sleep diary and questionnaires after each treatment phase. Which of the following best describes this study design?

    A. Case-control study

    B. Crossover study

    C. Cross-sectional study

    D. Prospective cohort study

    E. Randomized controlled trial

    Answer B: Crossover study. While this study is also a type of randomized controlled trial, the key feature is that the intervention is swapped between groups during the study period. Therefore, a crossover study is the most appropriate description of this study design.

Questions on Phases of Clinical Trials

33. A team of researchers are conduction a study to evaluate the safety and pharmacokinetics of a novel anti-inflammatory drug, Inflaxan. The drug is administered intravenously in increasing doses ranging from 1 to 50 mg/kg to 18 healthy volunteers. Blood samples are collected at regular intervals to determine the drug's half-life, absorption rate, and metabolite formation. Volunteers are closely monitored for side effects like allergic reactions, organ function abnormalities, and general tolerability. Inflaxan is well tolerated, with mild side effects such as transient headaches and fatigue, observed only at the highest doses. Which of the following best describes this type of study?

    A. Preclinical study

    B. Phase I clinical trial

    C. Phase II clinical trial

    D. Phase III clinical trial

    E. Phase IV clinical trial

    Answer: B. Phase I clinical trial. This study is not an animal study; it involved a small group of healthy volunteers and focused on safety testing. Therefore, it qualifies as a Phase I clinical trial.

34. To explore the potential of cetilistat, as a new anti-obesity drug, researchers conduct a study involving 85 individuals with obesity who have failed to lose weight with lifestyle interventions. The participants are randomized into groups receiving either a placebo or one of three different doses of cetilistat for 16 weeks. The primary outcomes include changes in body weight, body mass index (BMI), and waist circumference. Results indicate a significant dose-dependent reduction in weight and BMI with the new drug, though higher doses are associated with side effects like nausea and fatigue. Researchers find that the intermediate dose is the most promising for further investigation. Which of the following best describes this type of study?

    A. Preclinical study

    B. Phase I clinical trial

    C. Phase II clinical trial

    D. Phase III clinical trial

    E. Phase IV clinical trial

    Answer: C. Phase II clinical trial. This study involved a small group of affected individuals and focused on evaluating the treatment's efficacy and identifying side effects. Therefore, this is a Phase II clinical trial.

35. AXS-05, a new antidepressant is undergoing a clinical trial to determine its effectiveness in treating major depressive disorder compared to the current standard of care. 500 patients with moderate to severe depression are randomized into two groups: one group receives AXS-05, and the other group receives the current standard antidepressant. After six months, researchers evaluate improvement using standardized depression rating scales. AXS-05 shows comparable efficacy to the standard treatment but with fewer reported side effects, such as drowsiness and sexual dysfunction. Which of the following best describes this type of study?

    A. Preclinical study

    B. Phase I clinical trial

    C. Phase II clinical trial

    D. Phase III clinical trial

    E. Phase IV clinical trial

    Answer: D. Phase III clinical trial. In this study, a larger group of affected individuals is used to compare the treatment's efficacy with the standard of care. Therefore, this qualifies as a Phase III clinical trial.

36. A post-marketing evaluation is undertaken to assess the long-term effectiveness and side effects of a Semaglutide used in patients with Type 2 diabetes. The study includes 15,000 patients who use the drug for 18 months. While the drug maintains blood sugar control in most patients, liver enzyme elevations are noted in 48 individuals, prompting further investigations. The study suggests that patients with pre-existing liver conditions may require periodic liver function tests while on the medication. Which of the following best characterizes this type of study?

A. Phase I clinical trial

B. Phase II clinical trial

C. Phase III clinical trial

D. Phase IV clinical trial

E. Preclinical study

Answer: D. Phase IV clinical trial. Since this is a post-market study that monitors long-term side effects, it qualifies as a Phase IV clinical trial.

Questions on study parameters

37. An oncologist is conducting a prospective cohort study to examine the potential link between radiation exposure and the development of thyroid cancer in healthcare workers who are frequently exposed to radiation in medical settings. She follows a cohort of healthcare workers who work with radiation and a cohort of healthcare workers who do not, monitoring them for 10 years to assess the incidence of thyroid cancer in both groups. Which of the following would be the most appropriate measure of interest for this study?

A. Average radiation dose received by exposed workers

B. Incidence of thyroid cancer in each cohort

C. The number of thyroid ultrasounds performed in the exposed cohort

D. The rate of other cancers in both cohorts

E. The survival rate of those who develop thyroid cancer

Answer: B. Incidence of thyroid cancer in each cohort. The outcome of interest is the development of thyroid cancer, incidence of thyroid cancer in each cohort is the most appropriate measure.

Questions on selection of samples

38. A prospective cohort study aims to investigate the association between high dietary salt intake and the risk of developing hypertension in young adults. The exposed group consists of individuals who consume a high-sodium diet and do not have hypertension at baseline. Which of the following is the most appropriate comparison group for this study?

A. Young adults who consume a high-sodium diet and have hypertension

B. Young adults who consume a low-sodium diet and do not have hypertension

C. Young adults who consume a low-sodium diet and have hypertension

D. Young adults who consume a moderate-sodium diet and do not have hypertension

E. Young adults who consume a moderate-sodium diet and have hypertension

Answer: B. Young adults who consume a low-sodium diet and do not have hypertension. Since the outcome of interest is hypertension, participants should not have hypertension at the start of the study. Additionally, to compare the effects of high salt intake, participants with low-sodium consumption should be selected as comparison group.

39. A community is experiencing an outbreak of gastrointestinal illness linked to a possible contamination of the local water supply. Health officials conduct a case-control study to investigate the association between consuming water from the local supply and the development of gastrointestinal illness. The case group consists of individuals who have been diagnosed with gastrointestinal illness. Which of the following populations should be selected as the control group?

A. Individuals who do not have gastrointestinal illness and do not drink water from the local supply

B. Individuals who do not have gastrointestinal illness and drink water from the local supply

C. Individuals who do not have gastrointestinal illness, regardless of water consumption

D. Individuals who have gastrointestinal illness and drink water from the local supply

E. Individuals who have gastrointestinal illness, regardless of water consumption

Answer: C. Individuals who do not have gastrointestinal illness, regardless of water consumption. In a case-control study, the control group should not have the disease—in this case, gastrointestinal illness. Since the focus is on exposure status, the control group is selected based on the absence of the disease, regardless of the type of water consumption.

40. A study is conducted to evaluate the effectiveness of Aprocitentan (a dual endothelin A and B receptor antagonist), a new antihypertensive drug in reducing blood pressure among patients with stage 2 hypertension. A total of 150 patients are enrolled and randomly assigned to one of two groups, where one group receives the drug, and the other receives a placebo. The method of assigning patients to groups is most likely designed to accomplish which of the following?

    A. Ensuring that both groups have similar baseline blood pressure and demographics

    B. Ensuring that neither the researchers nor the participants know which treatment is received

    C. Ensuring that one group receives a higher dose than the other

    D. Guaranteeing that all participants receive the drug at some point in the trial

    E. Preventing one group from receiving any treatment at all

Answer: A. Ensuring that both groups have similar baseline blood pressure and demographics. The purpose of randomization is to control for both known and unknown confounders by making the two groups as similar as possible at baseline.

05 MEASURE OF ASSOCIATION AND THERAPEUTIC EFFICACY

In this chapter, we will explore various types of measures of association between risk factors and outcomes, how to choose the appropriate measure based on study design, and the methods for calculating these measures. Additionally, we will discuss other common measures of therapeutic efficacy.

LEARNING OUTCOME:

1. Choose an appropriate measure of association.
2. Calculate different types of measure of association.
3. Calculate measures of therapeutic efficacy.

5.1 REVIEW OF PREVIOUS CHAPTERS

5.1.1 Measure of Diseases Occurrence

A) **Incidence** refers to the number of new occurrences of a disease in a population over a specific period, representing the risk of developing the disease among the population at risk.

B) **Prevalence**, on the other hand, refers to the number of existing cases of a disease in a population at a given point in time.

Both incidence and prevalence are measures of disease burden, but they do not directly provide information about the relationship between exposure and disease.

5.1.2 Difference Between Risk and Odds

A) **Risk** is the probability of developing a disease or other health outcome over a specified study period and is a measure of incidence. To calculate risk, divide the number of affected subjects by the total number of subjects in the corresponding exposure group.

B) **Odds** refer to the ratio of the probability of an event occurring to the probability of it not occurring, expressed as $\left(\dfrac{P}{1-P} \right)$. Unlike risk, calculating odds does not involve the total number of people in the exposed and unexposed groups.

The probability of rolling a 1 on a single die is $\dfrac{1}{6}$, while the odds of rolling a 1 is $\dfrac{1}{5}$.

5.1.3 Study Designs

A) **Cross-Sectional Study**: A cross-sectional study is an observational study that assesses a population at a single point in time. It is commonly used to estimate disease prevalence and examine its association with specific risk factors.

B) **Case-Control Study**: A case-control study is an analytical observational design where participants are selected based on their disease status—either as cases (with the disease) or controls (without the disease). The exposure status is then compared between the two groups to assess the association between the disease and the exposure. In case-control studies, neither incidence nor prevalence can be directly measured.

C) **Cohort Study**: A cohort study is an observational analytic study design in which participants are categorized based on their exposure to a particular risk factor. They are then followed over time to assess the occurrence (i.e., incidence) of the outcome of interest in each group. The incidence of the outcome is compared between the exposed and non-exposed groups to estimate the association between the risk factors and outcomes.

D) **Clinical Trial**: A clinical trial is an experimental study where participants are prospectively assigned to two or more interventions (which may include a placebo or control treatment) to evaluate the effects of these interventions on outcomes of interest.

5.2 MEASURE OF ASSOCIATION

Clinical epidemiology goes beyond determining the frequency of disease occurrence by seeking to identify the causes of morbidity and mortality in human populations. To infer causal relationships, the existence of an association between diseases (dependent/outcome variables) and predisposing/risk factors (predictor/exposure variables) is explored by estimating measures of association.

The type of measure used depends on the study design and the nature of the data. In this section, we will focus on variables recorded in categorical form for both exposure and outcome. The association between two categorical variables, such as a categorical risk factor (e.g., smoker vs. nonsmoker) and a categorical outcome or disease (e.g., presence or absence of a condition like myocardial infarction), is calculated by properly formatting a 2×2 contingency table and applying the correct formula to determine the strength of association.

Outcome Risk factor	Disease (Present)	Disease (Present)	Total
Exposure (Present)	a	b	a+b
Exposure (Absent)	c	d	c+d
Total	a+c	b+d	a+b+c+d

Measures of association quantify the strength and direction of the relationship between exposure and outcome variables using ratios and differences. A ratio reflects the strength of the association between exposure and outcome, while a difference indicates the extent to which the outcome in the exposed group is associated with exposure.

5.2.1 Ratio-based Measures of Association

A) Relative Risk (RR)

Relative Risk is a measure used to assess the relationship between exposure to a specific risk factor or treatment and the likelihood of a particular outcome or disease. It compares the probability of developing the disease in individuals exposed to the risk factor with the probability in those who are not exposed. This measure is also known as the risk ratio or incidence ratio, and is frequently utilized in cohort studies and experimental research.

To calculate relative risk, the probability of an event (e.g., developing a disease) in the exposed group (e.g., the treatment group) is divided by the probability of the event in the unexposed group (e.g., the control group).

Calculation

RR= risk of disease in exposed / risk of disease in nonexposed

From 2 × 2 contingency table

$$RR = \frac{\dfrac{a}{(a+b)}}{\dfrac{c}{(c+d)}}$$

Interpretation

The RR may be interpreted as follows:

- RR <1.0 indicates that the exposure decreases the risk of disease.

- RR = 1.0 (null value) indicates that the exposure has no effect on the risk of disease.

- RR >1.0 indicates that the exposure increases the risk of disease.

An RR of 0.80 suggests that the exposure factor (e.g., treatment) reduces the risk of developing the outcome (e.g., disease) by 20%. Conversely, an RR of 3 indicates that the risk of the outcome is three times higher for those exposed to a specific risk factor compared to those who are not exposed.

The interpretation of relative risk (RR) depends on how the exposed and unexposed groups are defined. For instance, if a study examines the link between vaccination and the incidence of measles, participants are categorized based on their vaccination status: vaccinated or unvaccinated. The occurrence of measles within a specified period is then assessed in each group. The risk of the disease is compared between the exposed and unexposed groups to evaluate the association between the exposure (vaccination) and the disease.

If the exposed group is defined as the unvaccinated individuals and the unexposed group as the vaccinated individuals, the RR would be inverted.

B) Hazard Ratio (HR)

The Hazard Ratio (HR) is a statistical measure used in survival analysis to compare the risk of an event occurring at any given point in time between two groups. It quantifies the relative risk of the event happening in the treatment group compared to the control group over the study period. A HR greater than 1 indicates an increased risk in the treatment group, while a HR less than 1 indicates a decreased risk.

Calculation

The Hazard Ratio is calculated using the formula:

$$HR = \frac{\text{Hazard Rate in Treatment Group}}{\text{Hazard Rate in Control Group}}$$

To determine the hazard rates, survival data are analysed, often using methods such as the Cox proportional hazards model. The model estimates the hazard rates for each group and the ratio of these rates is used to derive the HR.

Application

Hazard Ratios are commonly used in clinical trials and epidemiological studies to assess the effectiveness of treatments or interventions. They help in understanding how different factors impact the time until an event occurs, such as disease progression or patient survival. For example, HR can be used to compare the time to recurrence of cancer between patients receiving a new drug versus a standard treatment.

C) Odds Ratio (OR)

The odds ratio (OR) is a statistical measure used in case-control studies to compare the likelihood of exposure between individuals with the disease (cases) and those without the disease (controls). Specifically, it reflects the odds of an outcome occurring in the presence of a particular exposure compared to the odds of the same outcome occurring in its absence.

While the odds ratio is useful, the relative risk (RR) often provides more clinical insight, as it shows how the presence or absence of risk factors influences the likelihood of developing a disease. However, RR cannot be calculated in case-control studies because these studies involve preselecting participants based on their disease status rather than sorting them into exposure groups and monitoring them over time to observe the incidence of new outcomes.

Diseases with very low incidence typically also have low prevalence. In case-control studies of rare diseases (generally with incidence below 10%), the odds ratio (OR) is often used to approximate the relative risk (RR), a concept known as the **rare disease assumption**. However, the accuracy of this approximation depends not only on prevalence but also on factors such as population stability and the control of confounding variables. Additionally, prevalence is influenced by factors like treatment outcomes, recovery rates, and mortality, which can introduce bias in etiological studies that rely on prevalent cases.

Calculation

OR = (odds of exposure in cases) / (odds of exposure in controls)
From 2 × 2 contingency table

$$OR = \frac{\dfrac{a}{c}}{\dfrac{b}{d}} = \frac{ad}{bc}$$

Interpretation

The Odds Ratio (OR) represents the odds of exposure among cases compared to controls. However, it is sometimes interpreted as the odds of developing a disease among those exposed versus those not exposed. The OR quantifies the relationship between exposure and disease, with a null value of 1 (OR=1).

- OR = 1.0 (null value) indicates that the odds of exposure among cases are the same as the odds of exposure among controls; therefore, exposure is not associated with the disease.

- OR ≠ 1.0 indicates that the odds of exposure are lower (ie, OR < 1) or higher (ie, OR > 1) among cases than among controls; therefore, exposure is associated with the disease.

D) Prevalence Ratio

Prevalence ratio is a ratio of 2 probabilities (i.e., prevalence) commonly used in cross-sectional studies to compare the prevalence of disease among exposed and unexposed groups of people.

Calculation

RR= prevalence of disease in exposed / prevalence of disease in nonexposed

Interpretation

As the exposure factor and outcome factors are collected simultaneously, this parameter represents mainly on association, not as risk factor.

E) Selecting an appropriate ratio measure based on study design

In observational studies that assess associations, four primary study designs are commonly employed: cross-sectional studies, case-control studies, prospective cohort studies, and retrospective cohort studies. The choice of the appropriate measure of association depends on the specific study design.

Cross-Sectional Studies: In cross-sectional studies, incidence cannot be measured because the study design does not involve tracking individuals over time. However, since the sample is drawn from the entire population at a single point in time, prevalence can be determined. The Prevalence Ratio is used as the measure of association, comparing the prevalence of disease between exposed and unexposed groups.

Case-Control Studies: In case-control studies, cases and controls are selected from a pool that may not accurately reflect the true frequency (prevalence) of disease in the population, leading to potential bias in prevalence estimates. Since cases already have the disease by definition, these studies do not track the development of disease over time. Consequently, risk cannot be measured, and Relative Risk (RR) cannot be calculated. Instead, the Odds Ratio is used as the measure of association.

Cohort Studies (Retrospective or Prospective): In cohort studies, the incidence or risk of disease can be measured by comparing the incidence rates between exposed and non-exposed individuals. The most commonly used measures of association in this design are Relative Risk (Risk Ratio/Incidence Ratio) or Relative Rate.

5.2.2 Difference-based Measures of association

Risk difference is the arithmetic difference between the risks, or cumulative incidence rates, of two groups: the exposed (or treatment) group and the unexposed (or control) group. Similarly, rate difference refers to the difference between the person-time incidence rates in these two groups. Depending on the direction of subtraction, the risk difference is referred to as either absolute risk reduction or absolute risk increase.

A) Absolute risk reduction (ARR)

Absolute Risk Reduction (ARR) is the difference in the risk (or event rate) of a negative outcome, such as disease incidence or death, between a control group and a treatment group. In other words, it represents the percentage of patients who benefit from the treatment compared to those in the control group (e.g., those receiving a placebo). ARR is a key measure for describing the efficacy of a treatment relative to a control.

Calculation

ARR = control rate - treatment rate

ARR represents the actual difference in event rates between the control and experimental groups. When the data is not presented in the standard format of a 2 × 2 contingency table, it's important to carefully select the appropriate values.

Interpretation

ARR = 0.20 indicates that 20% of patients did not develop an outcome as a result of having received treatment (eg. drug) rather than control (eg. placebo).

Application

ARR is used to calculate the number needed to treat (NNT). (see measures of therapeutic efficacy)

B) Relative Risk Reduction (RRR)

Relative risk reduction (RRR) measures how much a given treatment reduces the risk of an unfavourable outcome compared to the control group.

Calculation

$$\text{RRR} = \frac{\text{Risk}_{control} - \text{Risk}_{treatment}}{\text{Risk}_{control}} = \frac{\text{ARR}}{\text{Risk}_{control}}$$

Calculation of RRR from RR

$$RRR = 1 - RR$$

Calculation of Absolute Risk (Treatment)

When the Relative Risk Reduction (RRR) and the Absolute Risk (Control) are known, the Absolute Risk (Treatment) can be calculated using the following formula:

$$\text{Risk}_{treatment} = \text{Risk}_{control} - \left(\text{RRR x Risk}_{control} \right)$$

$$= \left(1 - \text{RRR} \right) \times \text{Risk}_{control}$$

Where:

- Absolute Risk (Treatment) is the event rate in the treatment group.
- Absolute Risk (Control) is the event rate in the control group.
- RRR (Relative Risk Reduction) is the proportional reduction in risk achieved by the treatment.

NB:
It is essential to use RRR as a decimal when using it in the calculation (e.g., 20% RRR should be used as 0.20)

Interpretation
RRR = 0.20 indicates that treatment (drug) offers a 20% reduction in outcome compared to control (placebo).

Application
RRR may overstate the effectiveness of an intervention. For example, a RRR of 20% occurs whether a drug decreases the incidence of a disease from 5% to 1% or from 25% to 5%. Clearly, the latter is of greater clinical significance.

C) Absolute risk increase (ARI)

Similarly, the Absolute Risk Increase (ARI) refers to the difference in the occurrence rate (risk) of an outcome (e.g., an adverse event) between the treatment group (e.g., those receiving a drug) and the control group (e.g., those receiving a placebo). To calculate ARI, subtract the adverse event rate in the control group from that in the treatment group. This subtraction is performed in the opposite direction compared to ARR.

Calculation
ARI = treatment rate – control rate

Application
Risk difference does not assume a causal relationship between exposure and outcome. It simply reflects how much of the outcome in the exposed group is associated with the exposure. If a causal relationship is assumed, the risk difference is equivalent to attributable risk (AR), and the rate difference corresponds to attributable rate. Additionally, these concepts are used to calculate measures of therapeutic effectiveness, such as the number needed to treat (NNT) and the number needed to harm (NNH).

D) Attributable Risk Percent (ARP or AR%)

Attributable Risk Percent (ARP) in the exposed population represents the proportion of excess risk that can be attributed to a specific risk factor. It quantifies the impact of a risk factor by indicating how much of the absolute risk of a disease in the exposed group is due to that exposure.

Calculation

$$ARP_{exposed} = \frac{Risk_{exposed} - Risk_{unexposed}}{Risk_{exposed}} \times 100\%$$

Since the relative risk (RR) is calculated as: $RR = \frac{Risk_{exposed}}{Risk_{unexposed}}$, ARP can also be determined using:

$$ARP_{exposed} = \frac{(RR-1)}{RR} \times 100\%$$

Interpretation

An ARP of 80% means that 80% of cases with the outcome (e.g., disease) in the exposed group can be attributed to the exposure. In other words, 80% of the disease occurrence in this group is caused by the exposure.

Application

If the exposure is eliminated, there would be an 80% reduction in disease incidence among the exposed group.

5.3 MEASURE OF THERAPEUTIC EFFICACY

Two key measures of therapeutic efficacy, the Number Needed to Treat (NNT) and the Number Needed to Harm (NNH), can be derived using the Absolute Risk Reduction (ARR) and Absolute Risk Increase (ARI).

5.3.1 Number Needed to Treat

The Number Needed to Treat (NNT) is the number of patients that need to be treated with a specific intervention to prevent one additional negative outcome (e.g., disease or death). It is a valuable indicator of a treatment's effectiveness.

NNT is calculated as the inverse of the Absolute Risk Reduction (ARR):

Calculation

$$NNT = \frac{1}{ARR}$$

Interpretation

NNTs are always rounded up to the nearest whole number. For example, if the ARR is 0.07, the NNT would be calculated as: $NNT = \frac{1}{0.07} \approx 14.3$. In this case, the NNT would be rounded up to 15. This means that approximately 15 patients with condition D (e.g., arthrosclerosis) need to be treated with medication M (eg. a new lipid lowering drug), in addition to standard therapy, to prevent one additional case of complication C (e.g., major cardiovascular adverse event) over a period of X years (according to the study duration).

Application

NNT is a useful tool for comparing the effectiveness of different treatments either within a single study or across similar studies (with comparable patient characteristics, control groups, and follow-up durations). A lower NNT indicates a more effective treatment since fewer patients need to be treated to prevent one additional negative outcome. The ideal NNT is 1, meaning that all treated patients benefit from the intervention.

5.3.2 Number Needed to Harm

Not all treatments are beneficial, and some can result in harm. The Number Needed to Harm (NNH) represents the number of patients who need to be treated before one additional adverse event occurs. It reflects the risk of harm caused by an intervention.

Calculation

NNH is calculated similarly to NNT, but using the Absolute Risk Increase (ARI) instead of ARR: $NNH = \frac{1}{ARI}$

Interpretation

For instance, an NNH of 50 means that approximately 50 patients would need to be treated with drug X for one patient to experience harm who otherwise would not have been harmed. The lower the NNH, the higher the risk of harm. An NNH of 1 would mean that every patient treated is harmed by the intervention.

Possible questions from this chapter

- Identify the appropriate measure of association
- Calculate Odds Ratio, Relative Risk and Relative Risk Reduction
- Calculate absolute risk, absolute risk reduction and absolute risk increase
- Calculate number needed to treat and number needed to harm
- Interpret number needed to treat and number needed to harm
- Calculate attributable risk percent
- Interpret the result findings

Questions on identification of appropriate measures of association

41. A team of researchers is conducting a study to determine if there is a relationship between environmental lead exposure and cognitive deficits in children. They select 30 children diagnosed with cognitive deficits from among all children who received preventative care at 10 local pediatric clinics over the past 3 years, as well as 60 children without the diagnosis. The mothers of both groups are interviewed about their residence in a known lead-contaminated geographic area. Which of the following measures of association is most appropriate for this type of study?

    A. Absolute risk reduction

    B. Hazard ratio

    C. Odds ratio

    D. Risk difference

    E. Prevalence ratio

    Answer: C. Odds ratio. Since this is a case-control study, the odds ratio is the most appropriate measure of association.

42. A study is designed to examine whether daily exercise reduces the risk of developing osteoporosis in postmenopausal women. Researchers recruited a group of women who exercised regularly and a group of women who did not, then followed both groups for 8 years to determine how many developed osteoporosis. What measure of association are the researchers most likely to use to compare the risk of osteoporosis between the two groups?

A. Incidence density

B. Odds ratio

C. Prevalence ratio

D. P-value

E. Relative risk

Answer: E. Relative Risk. Since this is a cohort study, the relative risk is the most likely measure of association to be used.

Questions on calculation of Odds Ratio (OR) and Relative Risk (RR)

43. A case-control study aims to investigate the relationship between regular consumption of fast food and the risk of developing type 2 diabetes in adults aged 30-50. The investigators collect data on fast food consumption among both the case group (those with type 2 diabetes) and the control group (those without diabetes). The results are shown below.

Fast food consumption	Type 2 Diabetes (+)	Type 2 Diabetes (-)	Total
Frequent	90	55	145
Rare	60	95	155
Total	150	150	300

Which of the following best represents the odds ratio of frequent fast-food consumption in adults with type 2 diabetes compared to those without diabetes?

A. 0.62

B. 1.60

C. 1.63

D. 2.59

E. 3.23

Answer: D. 2.59. $\mathrm{OR} = \dfrac{a \times d}{b \times c} = \dfrac{90 \times 95}{60 \times 95} = 2.59$

44. Researchers study whether eating a Mediterranean diet reduces the risk of developing type 2 diabetes. They found that 20 out of 200 type diabetic patients consume a Mediterranean diet, while 40 out of 150 non-diabetics consume a Mediterranean diet. What is the odds ratio for finding Mediterranean diet consumers among type 2 diabetes compared to non-diabetics?

A. (20 /60) / (180 /290)

B. (20 / 200) / (40 / 150)

C. (20 × 110) / (40 × 180)

D. (20 × 180) / (40 × 110)

E. (40 × 200) / (20 × 150)

Answer: C. (20 × 110) / (40 × 180). Constructing 2x2 table.

Mediterranean diet	Diabetes (+)	Diabetes (-)	Total
Consumer	20	40	60
Non- consumer	180	110	290
Total	200	150	350

45. A case-control study is conducted to explore the association between regular exposure to second-hand smoke and the risk of developing asthma in children. Researchers include 150 children diagnosed with asthma and 165 healthy children without asthma. The investigators assess second-hand smoke exposure in both groups. Among children with asthma, 30 were regularly exposed to second-hand smoke, while 15 of the healthy children had similar exposure. What is the estimated odds ratio of second-hand smoke exposure in children with asthma compared to those without asthma?

A. 0.5

B. 1.5

C. 2.0

D. 2.5

E. 4.0

Answer: D.2.5. From 2x2 table, $\text{OR} = \dfrac{a \times d}{b \times c} = \dfrac{30 \times 150}{15 \times 120} = 2.5$

Second hand smoke	Asthma (+)	Asthma (-)	Total
Exposed	30	15	45
Not exposed	120	150	270
Total	150	165	315

46. 45-year-old woman visits her physician to discuss the potential health risks associated with obesity. She is particularly concerned about her risk of developing type 2 diabetes. A recent cohort study compared the risk of developing type 2 diabetes in obese individuals with those of normal weight. The study reported that compared to individuals of normal weight, the relative risk (RR) of type 2 diabetes in obese individuals is 3.0. The patient asks how this compares to overweight individuals, who have an RR of 1.5. Based on the study, what is the relative risk of type 2 diabetes for obese individuals compared to overweight individuals?

A. 0.5

B. 1.0

C. 1.5

D. 2.0

E. 3.0

Answer: D. 2.0.

$$RR_{obesevsoverweight} = \frac{Risk_{obese}}{Risk_{overweight}} = \frac{\dfrac{Risk_{obese}}{Risk_{normal}}}{\dfrac{Risk_{overweight}}{Risk_{normal}}} = \frac{RR_{obese}}{RR_{overweight}} = \frac{3.0}{1.5} = 2.0$$

47. A study was conducted to assess the effect of regular physical exercise on the risk of developing type 2 diabetes in overweight adults. Over a 10-year follow-up period, 80 out of 350 adults who exercised regularly developed type 2 diabetes, while 140 out of 400 adults who did not exercise developed the condition. What is the relative risk of developing type 2 diabetes in adults who exercised regularly compared to those who did not?

A. (80×350) / (140×400)

B. (80×400) / (140×350)

C. (80/270) / (140/260)

D. (80/350) / (140/400)

E. (140/400) / (80/350)

Answer: D. (80/350) / (140/400). $RR_{exercise} = \dfrac{Risk_{exercise}}{Risk_{not\ exercise}} = \dfrac{80/350}{140/400}$

Questions on calculation of Relative Risk Reduction (RRR)

48. Researchers conducted a randomized controlled trial to assess the effectiveness of a new antiplatelet drug in reducing the risk of cardiovascular events (heart attacks, strokes) in patients with coronary artery disease. The study enrolled 200 participants, with 100 patients receiving the new drug and 100 patients receiving a placebo. After 2 years of follow-up, 10 patients in the new drug group experienced a cardiovascular event, while 15 patients in the placebo group experienced the same outcome. What is the relative risk reduction (RRR) for cardiovascular events among patients who received the new antiplatelet drug?

A. 0.05

B. 0.10

C. 0.15

D. 0.33

E. 0.67

Answer: D. 0.33. RRR = 1- RR; In this case is RR= $\dfrac{10/100}{15/100}$ = 0.67; RRR= 0.33

Questions on calculation of absolute risk, absolute risk reduction (ARR) and absolute risk increase (ARI)

49. A 55-year-old woman comes to the clinic for a routine visit. She is worried about her risk of developing osteoporosis as she ages, particularly since her mother had the condition. A recent cohort study assessed the impact of calcium intake on the development of osteoporosis over a 15-year period in 300 postmenopausal women. The results of the study are as follows:

Calcium intake	Developed osteoporosis	Did not develop osteoporosis	Total
Low	30	20	50
High	70	180	250
Total	100	200	300

Assuming this patient has a low calcium intake, what is her 15-year risk of developing osteoporosis?

A.   0.10

B.   0.28

C.   0.30

D.   0.50

E.   0.60

Answer: E. 0.60.

$$\text{Absolute risk}_{\text{low calcium intake}} = \frac{\text{No of cases among low Calcium intake}}{\text{Total people with low Calcium intake}} = \frac{30}{50} = 0.6$$

50. A randomized controlled trial is conducted to compare the effectiveness of a new antihypertensive drug versus standard care in reducing the risk of stroke in patients with hypertension. A total of 500 patients are enrolled in the study, with 250 randomly assigned to the new drug group and 250 to the standard care group. After 3 years of follow-up, the results are as follows:

Stroke Occurrence	Yes	No	Total
New drug	15	235	250
Standard care	30	220	250
Total	45	455	500

What is the absolute risk reduction (ARR) for stroke in patients treated with the new antihypertensive drug compared to those receiving standard care?

A. (30/250) - (15/250) = 0.06

B. (15/250) - (30/250) = -0.06

C. (30/250) - (15/250) / (30/250) = 0.5

D. (30/250) / (15/250) = 2.0

E. 1 / [(30/250) - (15/250)] = 16.67

Answer: A. **(30/250) - (15/250) = 0.06**. Absolute risk reduction (ARR) = $Risk_{standard\ care}$ - $Risk_{intervention}$ = (30/250) - (15/250) = 0.06.

51. A randomized controlled trial investigated the risk of drug-induced liver injury (DILI) in patients treated with a new antibiotic. A total of 1,200 patients were randomized to receive either the new antibiotic (600 patients) or a standard antibiotic (600 patients). The primary outcome was the incidence of DILI, defined as a significant elevation in liver enzymes. The study results showed 100 cases of DILI per 600 patients in the new antibiotic group, compared to 50 cases per 600 patients in the standard antibiotic group. Which of the following is the best estimate of the absolute risk increase (ARI) for DILI with the new antibiotic compared to the standard antibiotic?

A. (50/600) - (100/600)

B. (100/600) - (50/600)

C. (100/600) / (50/600)

D. (100/600) - (50/600) / (100/600)

E. $1 / [(100/600) - (50/600)]$

Answer: B. (100/600) - (50/600). Absolute risk reduction (ARI) = Risk_{new} drug - $\text{Risk}_{standard\ care}$ = $(100/600) - (50/600)$.

Questions on calculation of Number Needed to Treat (NNT) and Number Needed to Harm (NNH)

52. A study is conducted to evaluate the effectiveness of a new statin added to standard lipid-lowering therapy compared to standard therapy alone in preventing cardiovascular events (heart attacks or strokes) in patients with elevated cholesterol. After 4 years of follow-up, 85 of 100 patients in the new statin group had not experienced a cardiovascular event, compared to 80 of 100 patients in the standard therapy group. Based on these results, which of the following represents the approximate number of patients who need to be treated with the new statin to prevent one additional cardiovascular event over 4 years?

    A.   10
    B.   20
    C.   25
    D.   50
    E.   100

Answer: B. 20. Number needed to treat (NNT)

$$= \frac{1}{ARR} = \frac{1}{\left(\dfrac{85}{100}\right) - \left(\dfrac{80}{100}\right)} = \frac{1}{\dfrac{5}{100}} = 20$$

53. A physician research group is evaluating the efficacy of a new antihypertensive drug, Hypertrostat, in preventing strokes in patients with high blood pressure. The results of a 4-year, randomized, controlled study to evaluate the effectiveness of Hypertrostat are shown below.

	Number of patients treated with Hypertrostat	Number of patients treated with placebo
Stroke	15	30
No stroke	985	970

Based on these results, how many patients need to be treated with Hypertrostat to prevent one additional stroke?

A. 15

B. 30

C. 33

D. 50

E. 67

Answer: E. 67. Number needed to treat (NNT) =

$$\frac{1}{ARR} = \frac{1}{\left(\dfrac{30}{1000}\right) - \left(\dfrac{15}{1000}\right)} = \frac{1}{\dfrac{15}{1000}} = 67$$

54. A pharmaceutical company conducts a randomized, placebo-controlled study to evaluate the efficacy and safety of a new non-steroidal anti-inflammatory drug (NSAID) for patients with chronic osteoarthritis. The study reports that gastrointestinal (GI) bleeding occurred in 6% of patients taking the new NSAID compared to 2% in patients taking a placebo. Based on these results, how many patients need to be treated with the new NSAID to cause one additional case of GI bleeding?

A. 10

B. 15

C. 20

D. 25

E. 50

Answer: D. 25. Number needed to harm (NNH) = $\dfrac{1}{ARI} = \dfrac{1}{6\% - 2\%} = \dfrac{1}{4\%} = 25$

55. A randomized controlled trial is conducted to evaluate the safety of a new chemotherapy agent, Chemoblok, for treating advanced colorectal cancer. The trial compares the incidence of acute kidney injury (AKI) in patients receiving Chemoblok versus those receiving standard chemotherapy. The results are given below:

AKI	Chemoblok regimen	Standard chemotherapy
develop	20	10
do not develop	180	190

Based on these results, which of the following best represents the number needed to harm (NNH) for the Chemoblok regimen?

A. 10

B. 20

C. 30

D. 50

E. 100

Answer: B. 20.

Number needed to harm (NNH) = $\dfrac{1}{ARI} = \dfrac{1}{\left(\dfrac{20}{200}\right) - \left(\dfrac{10}{200}\right)} = \dfrac{1}{\dfrac{10}{200}} = 20$

Questions on calculation of Attributable Risk Percent (ARP)

56. A prospective cohort study is conducted to evaluate the association between high blood pressure and the risk of stroke in a population of middle-aged women. Over 15 years of follow-up, hypertensive women have 3 times the risk of developing stroke compared to women with normal blood pressure (relative risk = 3.0, 95% confidence interval = 1.8-4.2). According to the study results, what percentage of strokes in hypertensive women can be attributed to high blood pressure?

A. 33%

B. 50%

C. 67%

D. 75%

E. 90%

Answer: C. 67%.

Attributable risk percent ARP $= \dfrac{(RR-1)}{RR} \times 100\% = \dfrac{(3-1)}{RR3} \times 100\% = 67\%$

Questions on application (calculation of maximal acceptable risk)

57. Researchers are investigating the effectiveness of a new antihypertensive medication, BP-Plus, in reducing the risk of stroke. The stroke incidence in patients receiving standard therapy is 12%. Regulatory approval of BP-Plus requires a reduction in the stroke incidence by at least 25% compared to standard therapy. What is the maximal acceptable incidence of stroke for patients treated with BP-Plus?

    A. 6%

    B. 7%

    C. 8%

    D. 9%

    E. 10%

    Answer: D. 9% (25% reduction from 12%). The new drug, BP plus, will be approved if its associated incidence of stroke is decreased by at least 25% compared to incidence of stroke on standard therapy alone, which is given as 12%. As 25% of 12% is $0.25 \times 12\% = 3\%$, the maximum acceptable incidence of stroke is $12\% - 3\% = 9\%$. Another quick solution would be to state that the maximum acceptable incidence of stroke is 75% of 12%, which is $0.75 \times 12\% = 9\%$.

Questions on interpretation of result findings

58. Researchers conduct a randomized controlled trial to evaluate the effect of evolocumab, in reducing the risk of major adverse cardiovascular events in high-risk patients. The trial enrols patients with atherosclerosis and with high LDL cholesterol but without a prior ischemic event. Participants are randomly assigned to receive evolocumab or a placebo, and the incidence of major adverse cardiovascular events is measured for 5 years. The hazard ratio of major adverse cardiovascular events among patients receiving evolocumab compared to those receiving a placebo is 0.85 (95% confidence interval of 0.75–0.96). Which of the following is the most appropriate conclusion about the effect of evolocumab on the risk of major adverse cardiovascular events?

    A. Evolocumab has no significant effect on the risk of major adverse cardiovascular events

    B. Evolocumab reduces the risk of major adverse cardiovascular events by 85%

C. Taking evolocumab increases the risk of major adverse cardiovascular events by 15%

D. The risk of developing major adverse cardiovascular events in the evolocumab group is 0.85%

E. The risk of major cardiovascular events is reduced by 15% in patients taking evolocumab.

Answer: E. The risk of major cardiovascular events is reduced by 15% in patients taking evolocumab. The hazard ratio (HR) is similar to relative risk and is used in clinical trials. In this case, an HR of 0.85 indicates a (1 - 0.85) = 15% reduction in the risk of adverse cardiovascular (CVS) events.

59. A study compares the effectiveness of two new antihypertensive drugs, Drug X and Drug Y, in preventing strokes in elderly patients with hypertension. Patients are randomly assigned to receive Drug X, Drug Y, or placebo. The absolute risk reduction (ARR) of Drug X compared to placebo was found to be 0.10, while the ARR of Drug Y compared to placebo was 0.25. Which of the following statements comparing the effectiveness of Drugs X and Y is most appropriate?

A. Drugs X and Y require treating the same number of patients to prevent 1 additional stroke, so they are equally effective

B. Drug X requires treating fewer patients to prevent 1 additional stroke compared to Drug Y, so Drug X is less effective than Drug Y

C. Drug X requires treating fewer patients to prevent 1 additional stroke compared to Drug Y, so Drug X is more effective than Drug Y

D. Drug X requires treating more patients to prevent 1 additional stroke compared to Drug Y, so Drug X is less effective than Drug Y

E. Drug X requires treating more patients to prevent 1 additional stroke compared to Drug Y, so Drug X is more effective than Drug Y

Answer: D. Drug X requires treating more patients to prevent 1 additional stroke compared to Drug Y, so Drug X is less effective than Drug Y

STATISTICAL ANALYSIS

This chapter will discuss the principle of hypothesis testing, and different types of statistical analysis based on the type of variables.

LEARNING OUTCOME:

1. Understand the concept of hypothesis test.
2. Select an appropriate statistical test for analyzing research data.
3. Interpret the finding of correlation, statistical significance and p-value.
4. Deduct the level of statistical significance/ p-value from confidence interval.

In every research study, variables are typically summarized using measures of central tendency, and the relationship between exposure and outcome is assessed through measures of association. However, due to random variation, even an unbiased sample may not perfectly represent the entire population. Consequently, observed differences or associations could potentially arise by chance. The likelihood that an observed outcome is due to chance can be estimated through inferential statistics. Statistical testing of a research hypothesis enables the quantification of the risk of error when making inferences about a population based on sample data. This chapter provides an overview of the fundamental principles common to all statistical hypothesis tests and offers guidance on selecting the appropriate statistical test.

6.1 BASIS OF STATISTICAL REASONING

6.1.1 Hypothesis Testing

A statistical hypothesis is an initial assumption about population parameters (e.g., the mean values in two groups) or the relationship between variables within a population (e.g., the association between an exposure and a disease). Statistical tests are used to evaluate two competing hypotheses: the null hypothesis (H_0) and the alternative hypothesis (H_a). The null hypothesis (H_0) posits that there is no difference or no association between the variables, while the alternative hypothesis (H_a) suggests that there is a difference or an association.

Hypothesis testing may result in one of **FOUR** possible outcomes:

- **2 correct decisions:**

    - Fail to reject a true H_0 (ie, determine there is no correlation when one truly doesn't exist)

    - Reject a false H_0 (ie, determine there is a correlation when one truly exists)

- **2 incorrect decisions:**

    - Type I error: reject a true H_0 (ie, determine there is a correlation when one truly doesn't exist)

    - Type II error: fail to reject a false H_0 (ie, determine there is no correlation when one truly exists)

▼ **Table 6.1:** Type I (α) and Type II errors (β)

		True status	
		There is a true difference/ association (ie. H_0 is false)	There is NO true difference/ association (ie. H_0 is true)
Study result	Difference/ association calculated as statistically significant (ie. reject H_0)	Correctly conclude there is a difference/association (Confidence level)	**Falsely** conclude there is a difference/association (Type I (α) error)
	Difference/ association calculated as NOT statistically significant (ie. fail to reject H_0)	**Falsely** conclude there is **NO** difference/ association (Type II (β) error)	Correctly conclude there is **NO** difference / association (Power)

6.1.2   Type I and Type II Errors, Confidence level and Power

A **Type I error** occurs when a true null hypothesis (H_0) is incorrectly rejected, resulting in a false positive—finding a statistically significant difference when none actually exists. This leads the investigator to identify a relationship that does not exist. **Alpha (α)** represents the maximum probability of making a Type I error that a researcher is willing to accept, commonly referred to as the **significance level**. It is usually set by investigators as a threshold for rejecting the null hypothesis, often at 0.05, meaning there is a 5% chance of making a Type I error.

The **confidence level** is the complement of alpha, calculated as **(1 - α)**. It indicates the probability of correctly failing to reject a true null hypothesis, meaning the likelihood of not finding a statistically significant difference when none exists.

A **Type II error** occurs when a false null hypothesis is not rejected, resulting in a false negative—failing to detect a statistically significant difference when one actually exists. This leads to missing a true relationship. The probability of committing a Type II error is represented by **beta (β)**.

The **power of a test** is the probability of correctly rejecting a false null hypothesis, or in other words, detecting a true difference or correlation when one actually exists. It is calculated as **(1 - β)**, making it the complement of the Type II error rate. Power is typically set at 80%, meaning there is an 80% chance of detecting a difference if one truly exists. Power depends on several factors, including sample size and the magnitude of the difference between outcomes.

Lowering the significance level (**α**) reduces the probability of a Type I error, making the threshold for statistical significance more stringent and increasing the confidence level. However, this also decreases the statistical power of the study, meaning there is a higher chance of not detecting a statistically significant difference when one truly exists (i.e., an increased probability of a Type II error).

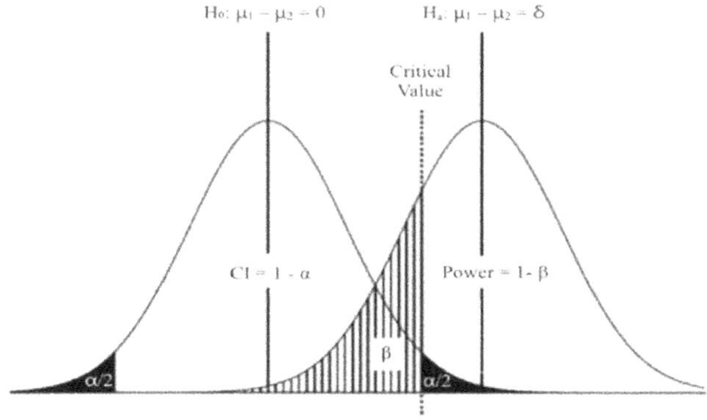

▲ **Figure 6.1:** Illustration of Hypothesis Testing: Type I and Type II Errors, Confidence Interval, and Statistical Power

6.1.3 P-value

To determine whether to reject the null hypothesis (H_0), researchers calculate the p-value. The **p-value** represents the probability of obtaining the observed results (or more extreme results) purely by chance, assuming H_0 is true. Typically, the p-value is compared to the significance level (α). If the p-value is less than α (e.g., $p < 0.05$), the result is considered statistically significant, suggesting an association between the variables or a difference in outcomes between groups with different exposures.

Conversely, a high p-value (e.g., ≥ 0.05) suggests that the sample result is close to the population value assumed under H_0, providing evidence in favour of H_0, meaning the null hypothesis might be correct and the results are not statistically significant.

It is important to note that the p-value reflects sampling variation (random variation) rather than bias (systematic variation) and is not linked to individual observations within the sample.

6.2 STATISTICAL TESTS FOR SIGNIFICANCE

In statistical analysis, the null hypothesis typically assumes that all groups are random samples from the same population, meaning their means are equal. The null hypothesis is rejected when at least two group means are found to be significantly different from one another.

6.2.1 Parametric Tests

A parametric test is a statistical test that makes specific assumptions about the parameters of the population distribution, such as the mean and variance. These tests assume that the data follows a certain distribution, typically normal, and are used to make inferences about population parameters based on sample data.

The scale of measurement of the dependent (e.g., outcome) and independent (e.g., exposures, risk factors) variables in a study determines the appropriate statistical test to use. Variables are generally classified as either qualitative (categorical) or quantitative (continuous) based on their measurement scale.

Qualitative variables (e.g., type of treatment, blood type) represent categories or groups, while quantitative variables (e.g., temperature, glucose levels) represent numerical values. Quantitative variables can sometimes be transformed into qualitative variables, such as categorizing temperature into "no fever" for values below 38°C (100°F) and "fever" for values of 38°C (100°F) or higher.

▼ **Table 6.2:** Decision making for statistical analysis (parametric tests) based on measurement scale of the variable

		Dependent variable	
		Qualitative (categorical)	Quantitative
Independent variable	Qualitative (categorical)	Chi-square, logistic regression*	*t* test, ANOVA, linear regression
	Quantitative	Logistic regression*	Correlation, linear regression
*Dependent variable must be dichotomous. ANOVA = analysis of variance.			

A) Chi-square Test

The Chi-square test assesses the relationship between two categorical variables, such as exploring the association between a predictor (e.g., presence or absence, or varying levels of exposure) and an outcome (e.g., the presence or absence of a disease). While Relative Risk (RR) or Odds Ratio (OR) can quantify the strength of this association, they do not account for the possibility that the observed results may be due to chance alone. To determine if the association is statistically significant, the p-value from the Chi-Square Test is used.

The Chi-square test specifically evaluates whether the distribution of observed frequencies differs from the expected frequencies under the null hypothesis of no association. It is used to test the "goodness of fit," or how well the observed data match the expected data.

Example: The Chi-square test can be used to explore the p-value in a study investigating the association between sex (e.g., "male" vs. "female") and myocardial infarction (e.g., presence vs. absence of myocardial infarction).

B) T-test

The mean difference is calculated to show the effect of a categorical predictor (e.g., treatment vs. no treatment) on a continuous outcome. T-tests are used to compare the mean of a quantitative variable between two groups and provide a p-value to determine statistical significance.

When comparing the means of two groups, there are two types of t-tests: the two-sample t-test (also known as the independent samples t-test) and the paired t-test.

The **two-sample t-test** is a statistical method often used to compare the means of an outcome variable between two independent groups.

Example: A two-sample t-test can be used to compare serum ferritin levels (a quantitative variable) between males and females.

The **paired t-test** compares the means of an outcome variable in two related groups, such as matched pairs or before-and-after treatment measurements.

Example: A paired t-test can be used to compare serum ferritin levels (a quantitative variable) before and after treatment with Silymarin in Thalassemia patients.

C) Analysis of Variance (ANOVA) test

Similar to the t-test, the ANOVA test compares the means between three or more independent groups in relation to the variability within groups (using the F-test) to determine whether there are statistically significant differences between group means. This test requires a categorical independent variable (e.g., exposure) that divides the study population into three or more groups, and a quantitative dependent variable (e.g., outcome) for which an average (e.g., mean) can be calculated. While it can be used to compare two groups, ANOVA is generally used for comparisons among three or more groups, as other methods like the two-sample t-test are more appropriate for comparing two groups. In fact, the two-sample t-test is a special case of the F-test in ANOVA, and the assumptions and resulting p-values for both tests are the same. When comparing the means of two groups, t-test and ANOVA results will be equivalent.

Example: ANOVA can be used to compare serum ferritin levels (a quantitative variable) in children (age 0-17), adults (age 18-59), and seniors (age 60 and above).

D) Regression analysis

Regression analysis can be either logistic or linear, depending on the type of outcome variable. If the outcome is binary (e.g., presence or absence of a condition), logistic regression is used. If the outcome is continuous (e.g., a numerical value), linear regression is applied.

Logistic regression is a method used to predict the probability of a binary outcome (e.g., presence or absence of disease). When multiple independent variables, either continuous or categorical, are included in the prediction model, it is referred to as multiple logistic regression.

Example: Logistic regression can be used to predict the probability of developing pancreatic cancer based on factors such as alcohol consumption, tobacco use, and charred food consumption.

Linear regression, on the other hand, models the linear relationship between a dependent variable and one or more independent variables. The dependent variable must be continuous, while the independent variables can be either continuous or categorical.

Example: Linear regression can be used to analyse the relationship between the number of cigarettes smoked per day and the number of yearly hospitalizations in COPD patients, described by a trend line.

E) Correlation

Correlation analysis assesses whether a linear relationship exists between two variables. For example, it can be used to evaluate the linear relationship between hours of sleep and an irritability score. Unlike linear regression, correlation provides a single number that describes the strength and direction of the association. The **Pearson correlation coefficient (r)** measures the strength and direction of the linear relationship between two quantitative (continuous) variables.

Scatter plots are useful tools for basic data analysis. When a linear association exists between two variables, the correlation coefficient (r) mathematically describes how well a line of best fit (red in the figure) corresponds to the plotted data points. The value of r ranges from -1 to +1, capturing two key aspects of the association: strength and polarity. The closer the r value is to the margins (-1 or +1), the stronger the association.

Strength:
when r values are close to -1 or 1, the linear relationship is strong;
when r values are close to 0, the linear relationship is weak.

Direction:
when r < 0, the linear relationship is negative and one variable increases as the other decreases;
when r > 0, the linear relationship is positive and both variables increase and decrease together.

It's important to note that the value of r is not the same as the slope of the line of best fit. For example, even with a strong positive association (r = +1), the slope of the line could vary (e.g., 0.2, 5.5, or any positive value). A value of r = -0.2 indicates a weak negative association, meaning there is more variation around the line of best fit.

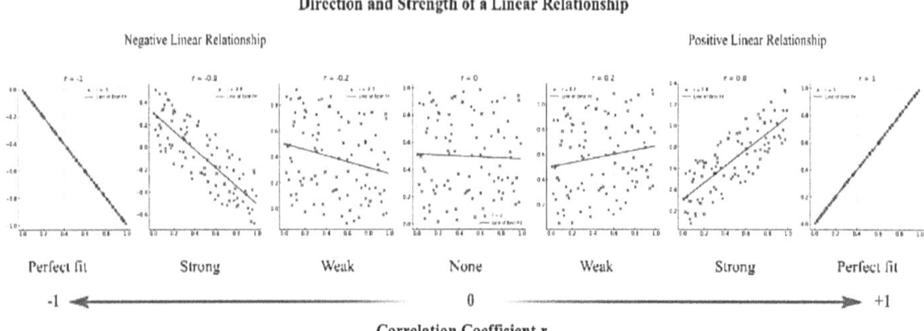

▲ **Figure 6.2:** Direction and Strength of a linear relationship

While correlation may involve a dependent and an independent variable, it does not imply causality. A statistically significant linear relationship (with a p-value below a certain threshold) also does not indicate causation. In other words, even if two variables are significantly correlated, one does not necessarily cause the other to change—correlation does not equal causation.

F) Meta-analysis

A meta-analysis is an epidemiological method that combines data from multiple studies, typically using quantitative statistical techniques to analyze the results. Ideally, it focuses on high-quality randomized controlled trials to provide an overall estimate of the effect of an exposure on a particular outcome. By pooling data, meta-analysis increases the statistical power beyond what individual studies can offer. While single studies may produce inconclusive results, combining data from several trials can often reveal significant benefits.

6.2.2 Non-parametric Tests

A non-parametric test is a type of statistical test that does not assume the data follows a specific distribution, such as the normal distribution. These tests are often used when the data does not meet the assumptions required for parametric tests, such as normality, or when the sample size is small. Non-parametric tests are also suitable for ordinal data or ranked data and can be more robust when dealing with outliers or skewed distributions. Common non-parametric tests include the Mann-Whitney U test, Wilcoxon signed-rank test, and Kruskal-Wallis test.

A) Mann-Whitney U Test

The Mann-Whitney U test compares two independent groups when the dependent variable is ordinal or continuous, but does not meet the assumption of normality. It is commonly employed to compare the median values between two groups. This test serves as the non-parametric alternative to the independent t-test.

Example: Comparing the effectiveness of two different treatments on pain scores where the data is not normally distributed.

B) Wilcoxon Signed-Rank Test

The Wilcoxon Signed-Rank test compares two related or paired groups, especially when the data is ordinal or continuous but does not follow a normal distribution. It is ideal for repeated measures or matched pairs data, such as pre-test and post-test comparisons. This test is appropriate when assessing median differences between two paired observations and serves as the non-parametric alternative to the paired t-test.

Example: Comparing blood pressure levels before and after an intervention in the same group of patients.

C) Kruskal-Wallis Test

The Kruskal-Wallis test compares more than two independent groups when the data is ordinal or continuous and does not follow a normal distribution. This test is suitable if you want to determine whether there are significant differences in the medians across three or more groups and serves as the non-parametric alternative to the one-way ANOVA.

Example: Comparing patient satisfaction scores across three different hospitals where the data is skewed.

▼ **Table 6.2:** Decision making for statistical analysis (non-parametric tests) based on measurement scale of the variable

	Parametric Tests	Non-parametric Test
Compare means of 2 independent groups	Independent t-test (2 sample t-test)	Mann-Whitney U Test
Compare means of 2 related groups	Paired t-test	Wilcoxon Signed-Rank Test
Compare means of more than 2 independent groups	ANOVA	Kruskal-Wallis Test

6.2.3   Confidence Intervals (CI) and Statistical Significance

In all studies, a null hypothesis is tested, but the null value differs depending on the type of outcome. For categorical outcomes (such as relative risk (RR) or odds ratio (OR)), the null value is 1, which means no difference in risk between the groups (RR/OR = 1). For continuous outcomes (like mean differences), the null value is 0, indicating no difference between the group means. Confidence intervals provide a range of plausible values for an unknown parameter (e.g., the difference between two mean systolic blood pressures). If the CI does not include the null value, the result is statistically significant, with a p-value < 0.05. However, if the CI crosses the null value, the result is not statistically significant.

6.2.4   Statistical Significance and Clinical Significance

Statistical significance does not always equate to clinical relevance. With a large sample size, even small differences can become statistically significant due to the increased power of the study. However, the actual effect size may be minimal and of little practical importance. For example, a study might find a statistically significant reduction in systolic blood pressure (SBP) following cocoa intake. While this result may be statistically significant, the clinical significance could be limited if the absolute decrease in SBP is only around 2 mm Hg, a reduction that may not have a meaningful impact on patient health outcomes.

Possible questions from this chapter

- Identify the appropriate null hypothesis
- Interpret significance and power, type I error, type II error
- Select an appropriate analysis method
- Identify and interpret correlation coefficient
- Interpret p value, confidence interval and level of significance
- Interpret the study result

Questions on Hypothesis test and underlying principles

60. A randomized controlled trial is conducted to determine the effect of a new drug in reducing the risk of deep vein thrombosis (DVT) in post-operative patients. A total of 300 patients are randomly assigned to receive either the new drug or a placebo. The incidence of DVT is compared between the two groups over a 6-month period. Which of the following is the most appropriate null hypothesis for this study?

A. Hazard ratio is equal to 1

B. Hazard ratio is not equal to 1

C. Odds ratio is equal to 1

D. Odds ratio is not equal to 1

E. Relative risk is equal to 1

F. Relative risk is not equal to 1

Answer: A. Hazard ratio is equal to 1. Since this is a randomized controlled trial, the hazard ratio would be the appropriate measure, especially if time-to-event (DVT) is considered, and the null hypothesis states that the hazard ratio is equal to 1.

61. A clinical trial is planned to evaluate the efficacy of **Orlistat**, a lipase inhibitor for weight loss in obese patients. Researchers want to ensure that they can detect a meaningful difference in weight loss between the drug and placebo groups if such a difference exists. Which of the following factors should they aim to maximize in order to increase the likelihood of detecting this difference?

A. α

B. β

C. Type I error

D. Type II error

E. $1 - \beta$

Answer: E. $1 - \beta$. In order to increase the likelihood of detecting the difference, power must be increased, which is $1 - \beta$.

62. A clinical trial examines the effectiveness of suzetrigine, a new pain relief medication. Researchers find that the average pain score for patients taking the suzetrigine is 3 on a scale of 1 to 10, compared to an average score of 5 for those taking a placebo. The p-value for the observed difference is reported as 0.03. Furthermore, there is a 15% chance of incorrectly concluding that there is no difference when there actually is one. What is the power of the study?

    A. 0.15

    B. 0.20

    C. 0.70

    D. 0.85

    E. 0.95

    Answer: D. 0.85. 15% chance of incorrectly concluding that there is no difference when there actually is one represents a β value of 0.15, meaning the power of the study is 0.85 (or 85%).

63. In a clinical trial assessing the effectiveness of a new antihypertensive medication, researchers found a significant reduction in systolic blood pressure. They state, "The reduction in systolic blood pressure was statistically significant, with a probability of observing this result due to by chance is 1% with a 20% chance of not rejecting the null hypothesis when there is one in reality. Given this scenario, which of the following correctly represents the p-value and the power of the test conducted in the study?

    A. p-value of 0.01; power of 0.80

    B. p-value of 0.01; power of 0.90

    C. p-value of 0.02; power of 0.80

    D. p-value of 0.02; power of 0.90

    E. p-value of 0.05; power of 0.80

    F. p-value of 0.05; power of 0.90

    Answer: A. p-value of 0.01 and a power of 0.80. 1% probability of observing the result due to by chance implies p-value is 0.01. The 20% chance of not rejecting the null hypothesis when there is one in reality represents a β value of 0.2, meaning the power of the study is 0.8 (or 80%).

64. In a study evaluating the effects of Aprocitentan, an endothelin receptor antagonist used as an antihypertensive drug, researchers are planning to recruit participants. They want to make sure they have enough participants to confidently determine if the medication leads to a statistically significant reduction in blood pressure compared to a placebo. What should the researchers focus on to ensure they have sufficient statistical power?

A. Decreasing confidence level

B. Increasing α

C. Increasing β

D. Minimizing variability in measurements

E. Reducing sample size

Answer: D. Minimizing variability in measurements. Power is the ability of a study to detect a true effect if it exists. It depends on several factors, including the sample size, effect size, significance level (α), and variability in the data. Minimizing variability in measurements improves the precision of the study, making it easier to detect a true difference between the treatment (Aprocitentan) and placebo, thus increasing statistical power.

A. Decreasing confidence level: This would reduce confidence in the results, not necessarily increase power.

B. Increasing α: While increasing α (the probability of a Type I error) could technically increase power, it would also increase the risk of falsely rejecting the null hypothesis, which is generally undesirable.

C. Increasing β: β is the probability of a Type II error (failing to detect a true effect). Increasing β would actually decrease power.

E. Reducing sample size: This would reduce the study's power, as a smaller sample size makes it harder to detect a true effect.

Therefore, minimizing variability in measurements is the best option for ensuring sufficient statistical power.

65. A clinical trial is conducted to evaluate the effectiveness of Orlistat upon weight reduction compared to a placebo. The researchers initially set the significance level (alpha) at 0.05. After reviewing the literature, they decide to change the alpha level to 0.001 to minimize the risk of false positives. What is the most likely consequence of this decision?

A. The chance of a Type I error will increase

B. The probability of a Type II error will decrease

C. The study will be less likely to declare a treatment effect even if it exists

D. The study will have less confidence in its significant findings

E. The study's statistical power will increase

Answer: C. The study will be less likely to declare a treatment effect even if it exists. Lowering the α level reduces the risk of Type I errors (false positives), meaning the threshold for declaring a result significant becomes stricter. This makes the study less likely to detect a treatment effect, even if one actually exists, increasing the likelihood of a Type II error (false negatives). Lowering alpha also decreases statistical power (the ability to detect a true effect).

Questions on selection of analysis methods

66. A study was conducted to estimate the association between serum level of fibrinogen and ischemic stroke. Cases were identified as those having ischemic stroke and controls were those with no CVD event. Plasma fibrinogen level was measured and categorized into normal and high. The following table summarizes the findings:

Fibrinogen level	Ischemic stroke (Yes)	No CVD event (No)	Total
High	45	55	100
Low	15	85	100
Total	60	140	200

Which statistical test is most appropriate to assess the association between smoking status and lung cancer occurrence in this study?

A. Analysis of variance

B. Chi-square test

C. Correlational analysis

D. Meta-analysis

E. Two-sample t-test

Answer: B. Chi-square test. Since both the outcome and predictor variables are categorized into two groups, the chi-square test is appropriate.

67. A study is conducted to compare the effectiveness of morphine and methadone in patients with chronic pain. Group A, which received Morphine, reports a mean pain score of 8.5 (on a scale of 0-10) with a standard deviation of 1.0. Group B, which received Methadone, reports a mean pain score of 7.7 with a standard deviation of 1.2. Which statistical method should be used to compare the mean pain scores of these two groups?

A. ANOVA

B. Chi-square test

C. Paired t-test

D. Regression analysis

E. Two-sample t-test

Answer: E. Two-sample t-test. In this study, the outcome is the pain score (a continuous variable) between two independent groups (morphine and methadone). A two-sample t-test, also known as an independent t-test, is the appropriate method for analysis.

68. A clinical trial is conducted to evaluate the effectiveness of a new cognitive-behavioral therapy (CBT) program for reducing anxiety levels in patients with generalized anxiety disorder. Researchers measure anxiety levels using a standardized scale before and after the therapy in the same group of patients. The scores before therapy show a mean of 28 with a standard deviation of 5, and the scores after therapy show a mean of 22 with a standard deviation of 4. Which statistical test should be used to compare the pre-therapy and post-therapy anxiety scores?

A. Analysis of variance

B. Chi-square test

C. Independent t-test

D. Paired t-test

E. Regression analysis

Answer: D. Paired t-test. The outcome (anxiety level) is measured on a continuous scale, and the mean anxiety levels are compared before and after the therapy. Since the same patients are involved, a paired t-test is the appropriate method for analysis.

69. A nutritionist conducts a study to evaluate the effects of three different diets (Diet A, Diet B, and Diet C) on weight loss over 12 weeks. Participants are randomly assigned to one of the three diet groups, with 50 participants in each group. At the end of the study, the weight loss of each participant is measured. Which statistical method is most appropriate for comparing the mean weight loss among the three diet groups?

A. Analysis of variance

B. Chi-square test

C. Paired t-test

D. Simple linear regression

E. Wilcoxon rank-sum test

Answer: A. Analysis of variance. This study compares the mean weight (dependent – continuous variable) between 3 different groups, ANOVA is the most appropriate test.

70. A hospital research team is conducting a study to evaluate how different lifestyle factors influence cholesterol levels in adults aged 30-60. The study aims to assess the impact of two independent variables: daily sugar intake (in grams) and weekly exercise duration (in hours) on LDL cholesterol levels (mg/dL), while adjusting for age, BMI, and smoking status. Which statistical technique is most appropriate for determining the association between the independent variables and LDL cholesterol levels, while accounting for the control variables?

A. Analysis of variance

B. Chi-square test

C. Logistic regression

D. Meta-analysis

E. Regression analysis

Answer: E. Regression analysis. Regression analysis is the preferred method for examining the association between a continuous outcome (e.g., LDL cholesterol level) and independent variables, while adjusting for known confounders

71. A medical researcher is interested in investigating the relationship between the number of hours of weekly physical activity and high-density lipoprotein cholesterol (HDL-c) levels in adults aged 30-70. Participants are surveyed about their average hours of weekly physical activity, and their cholesterol levels are measured through blood tests. To determine the strength of association between physical activity and cholesterol levels, which statistical method should be used?

A. Analysis of variance

B. Chi-square test

C. Correlation analysis

D. Paired t-test

E. Two-sample t-test

Answer: C. Correlation analysis. To measure the strength of the association between two continuous variables (hours of physical activity and HDL-cholesterol level), correlation analysis is appropriate.

Questions on correlation coefficient

72. A nutritionist is studying the relationship between fruit and vegetable intake and body mass index (BMI) among a group of 300 adults. The researcher finds that as fruit and vegetable intake increases, BMI tends to decrease. The correlation analysis shows a strong relationship between the two variables. Based on this information, which of the following statements best describes the associated correlation coefficient?

    A. It is negative and probably closer to 0 than to -1

    B. It is negative and probably closer to -1 than to 0

    C. It is positive and probably closer to 0 than to 1

    D. It is positive and probably closer to 1 than to 0

    Answer: B. It is negative and probably closer to -1 than to 0. The finding indicates that as fruit and vegetable intake increases, BMI tends to decrease, demonstrating a negative association. A strong negative association would result in a correlation value closer to -1 than to 0.

73. A researcher examines the relationship between exercise frequency (measured in hours per week) and cholesterol levels (measured in mg/dL) in a group of 120 adults. After plotting the data, the researcher observes that as exercise frequency increases, cholesterol levels tend to decrease. When the exercise frequency is plotted against cholesterol level, the following plot is obtained.

    Based on the plot, the correlation coefficient between the two variables is closest to which of the following values?

    A. +0.7

    B. +0.3

    C. 0

    D. -0.5

    E. -0.9

    Answer: E. -0.9. The graph shows a negative trend, and the data points are closely clustered, indicating a strong relationship. Therefore, the most likely correlation coefficient is -0.9.

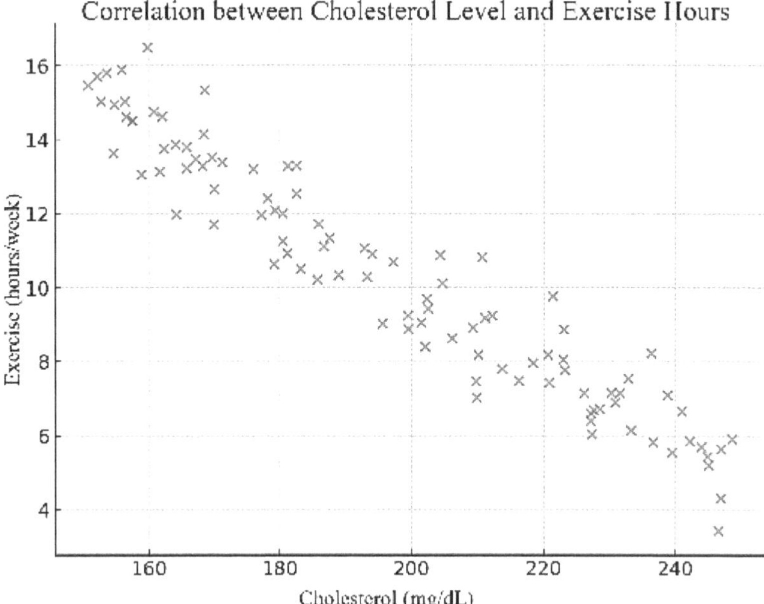

74. A study is conducted to evaluate the relationship between daily screen time (in hours) and academic performance (measured by GPA) among high school students. After analysing the data, researchers find a correlation coefficient of r = -0.58 (p < 0.01) between screen time and GPA. What is the most accurate interpretation of these results?

A. An increase in screen time causes a statistically significant decrease in academic performance.

B. Increased screen time has no impact on academic performance among high school students.

C. Increased screen time leads to higher GPAs among students.

D. There is a statistically significant negative linear relationship between screen time and academic performance.

E. There is a statistically significant positive linear relationship between screen time and academic performance.

Answer: D. There is a statistically significant negative linear relationship between screen time and academic performance. With r = -0.58, the relationship is negative, and since p < 0.01, it is statistically significant, D is the correct answer.

Questions on p-value, confidence interval and statistical significance

75. A randomized controlled trial was conducted to assess the effectiveness of Aprocitentan, an endothelin receptor antagonist, in reducing blood pressure compared to a placebo. The study reports a mean difference in systolic blood pressure of 10 mmHg (95% confidence interval: 3-17 mmHg) between the medication group and the placebo group. Which of the following p-values is most consistent with these results?

    A. 0.01

    B. 0.04

    C. 0.07

    D. 0.10

    E. 0.15

    Answer: B. 0.04. Since the 95% confidence interval is 3–17 mmHg, it does not cross the null value of 0 mmHg, indicating statistical significance ($p < 0.05$). However, the interval is relatively wide, suggesting that the p-value is likely closer to 0.04 rather than 0.01.

76. In a double-blind, placebo-controlled trial on the antihypertensive treatment effect of a quadruple single-pill combination, researchers reported the between-group difference in diastolic blood pressure was -6.0 mmHg with a 95% confidence interval of −9.7 to −2.2 mmHg. Which of the following statements best represents the results of this trial?

    A. The difference is not statistically significant

    B. The drug has no effect on diastolic blood pressure

    C. The drug increases diastolic blood pressure

    D. The drug significantly lowers diastolic blood pressure

    E. The p-value is greater than 0.05

    Answer: D. The drug significantly lowers diastolic blood pressure. Since the 95% confidence interval is -9.7 to -2.2 mmHg, it does not contain the null value of 0 mmHg, indicating statistical significance ($p < 0.05$).

77. A study investigating the impact of dietary sodium on blood pressure conducted several trials. The results for each trial comparing the mean blood pressure of individuals on a low-sodium diet versus a regular sodium diet are as follows:

Study	Mean BP $_{\text{Low-Sodium}}$ – Mean BP $_{\text{Control}}$ (mm Hg) [95% CI]
1	-4.5 [-6.2, -2.8]
2	0.3 [-1.5, 2.1]
3	-3.0 [-5.5, -0.5]
4	-1.5 [-3.2, 0.2]
5	-2.1 [-4.0, -0.2]
6	0.5 [-0.5, 1.5]
Total	-1.8 [-2.5, -1.0]

Based on this data, which of the following conclusions is most appropriate?

A. A higher mean blood pressure was observed in the low-sodium groups overall.

B. Low-sodium diets should be recommended for blood pressure management.

C. Low-sodium intake was associated with a statistically significant decrease in blood pressure.

D. Studies 2 and 6 showed a statistically significant increase in blood pressure.

E. There was no statistically significant change in blood pressure overall.

Answer: C. Low sodium intake was associated with a statistically significant decrease in blood pressure. Answer D is incorrect because the confidence interval contains the null value, indicating that these studies are not statistically significant. However, when the data were pooled, the difference in mean blood pressure between the low-sodium group and the control group was 1.8 mmHg lower. The confidence interval for this difference does not include the null value of 0, making the finding statistically significant.

Questions on interpretation of study finding

78. A clinical trial investigates the effect of a high-protein diet versus a standard diet on muscle mass in older adults. Researchers recruit 200 participants aged 65 and older, randomizing them into a high-protein diet group (30% of daily calories from protein) or a standard diet group (15% of daily calories from protein) in a 1:1 ratio. After 6 months, the high-protein group showed an increase in muscle mass compared to the standard diet group, with a mean difference of +2.8 kg ($p = 0.03$, predetermined significance level = 0.05). Which of the following is the most accurate interpretation of the results of this study?

A. The observed mean difference in muscle mass of +2.8 kg is not statistically significant

B. The probability of observing a mean difference in muscle mass of +2.8 kg is 0.03

C. There is a 3% chance of observing a mean difference in muscle mass of at least +2.8 kg when no difference between groups is assumed

D. There is a 3% chance that an older adult on a high-protein diet will have a muscle mass increase of at least +2.8 kg at 6 months

E. E. There is a 3% chance that the mean difference in muscle mass is biased in favour of the high-protein diet group

Answer: C. There is a 3% chance of observing a mean difference in muscle mass of at least +2.8 kg when no difference between groups is assumed. The p-value is a statistical measure that helps you understand the significance of your results. Specifically, it tells you the probability of getting a sample result as extreme as (or more extreme than) the one you observed, assuming the null hypothesis is correct.

In this case, the given p-value = 0.03; therefore, there is a 3% chance (ie, 0.03) of observing a mean difference in muscle mass (ie, sample estimate) of at least +2.8 kg between the high protein diet and the standard diet when no difference between groups is assumed (ie, null hypothesis is assumed to be true)

PROPERTIES OF A SCREENING TEST

This chapter discusses the measures used to assess the quality of a screening test and how they are applied in clinical practice.

LEARNING OUTCOME:

1. Differentiate between precision (reliability) and accuracy (validity).
2. Calculate common performance indicators of a test (Sensitivity, Specificity).
3. Calculate the likelihood indicators (PPV, NPV).
4. Discuss the factors effecting the test parameters.
5. Interpret the findings of test parameters.
6. Interpret the ROC curve.

The ultimate aim of an investigative test is to detect diseases for early diagnosis and prompt treatment. If a screening test misses an infectious disease, controlling the spread of the infection becomes impossible. Similarly, on an individual level, if a diagnostic test fails to detect the disease, the patient may not receive appropriate treatment. Therefore, the performance characteristics of a test play a crucial role in both screening and diagnosis.

7.1 PRECISION AND ACCURACY

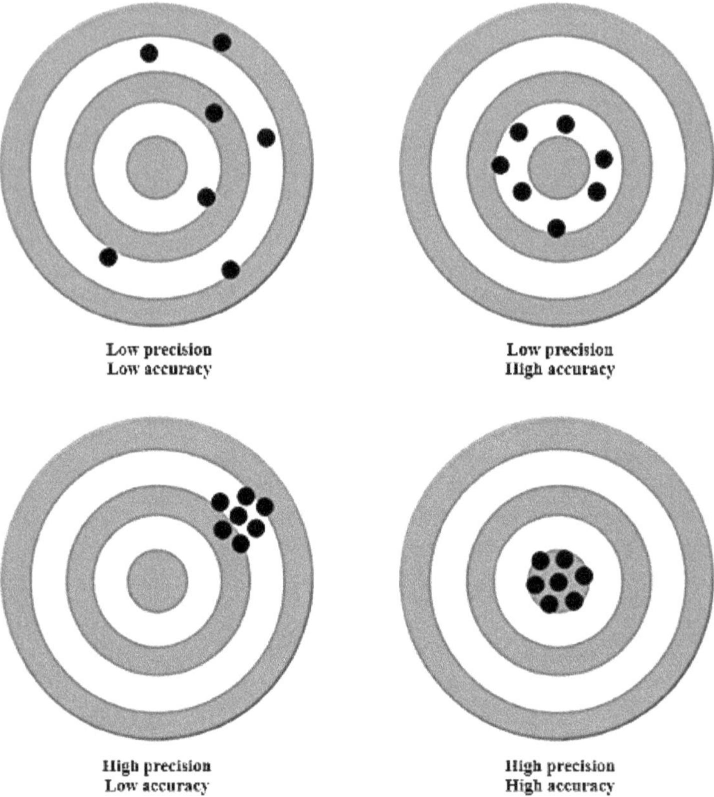

▲ **Figure 7.1:** Precision and Accuracy

Precision (or reliability) refers to a test's ability to consistently produce identical or similar results with repeated measurements.

Accuracy (or validity) refers to a test's ability to measure what it is intended to measure. For a new test to be considered accurate, its results should align closely with those of a gold standard.

For example, if repeated measurements, such as a person's blood pressure or blood sample, yield nearly identical values, the test is considered highly precise. However, high precision does not necessarily indicate accuracy. A diagnostic device can be precise but still provide incorrect results if those values are far from the true or actual value.

7.2 COMMON PERFORMANCE PARAMETERS OF A TEST

A diagnostic test may result in one of **FOUR** possible outcomes:

	Diseased	Disease-free
Positive Test Result	True positives (TP)	False positive (FP)
Negative Test Result	False Negative (FN)	True negative (TN)

7.2.1 Sensitivity (Positivity Among Diseased Individuals)

It is the probability that a diseased patient has a positive result. (The probability of an individual testing positive given the presence of disease)

Calculation

$$\text{sensitivity} = \frac{\text{diseased with positive test}}{\text{all diseased}}$$

$$= \frac{\text{True Positives (TP)}}{\text{True Positives (TP)} + \text{False negatives (FN)}}$$

Sensitivity measures a test's ability to correctly identify individuals with the disease. A test with high sensitivity ensures that most patients with the condition will test positive, making a negative result useful for ruling out the disease (SnNOut).

7.2.2 Specificity (Negativity Among Healthy Individuals)

It is the probability that a disease-free individual has a negative result. (The probability of an individual testing negative given the absence of disease)

Calculation

$$\text{specificity} = \frac{\text{disease} - \text{free with negative test}}{\text{all disease} - \text{free}}$$

$$= \frac{\text{True Negatives (TN)}}{\text{True Negatives (TN)} + \text{False Positives (FP)}}$$

Specificity measures a test's ability to correctly identify individuals without the disease. A highly specific test has a low rate of false positives, making it valuable for confirmation. A test with high specificity, most healthy individuals will receive a negative result, making a positive result useful for ruling in the presence of the disease (SpPIn).

7.2.3 False Positive Rate

It is the probability that a disease-free individual has a positive result. (The probability of an individual testing positive given the absence of disease)

Calculation

$$\text{False positive rate} = \frac{\text{disease} - \text{free with positive test}}{\text{all disease} - \text{free}}$$

$$= \frac{\text{False Positives}\left(\text{FP}\right)}{\text{True Negatives}\left(\text{TN}\right) + \text{False Positives}\left(\text{FP}\right)}$$

7.2.4 False Negative Rate

It is the probability that a diseased has a negative result. The probability of an individual testing negative given the presence of disease)

Calculation

$$\text{False negative rate} = \frac{\text{diseased with negative test}}{\text{all diseased}}$$

$$= \frac{\text{False Negative}\left(\text{FN}\right)}{\text{True Positives}\left(\text{TP}\right) + \text{False negatives}\left(\text{FN}\right)}$$

7.2.5 Positive Predictive Value (PPV)

It is the probability that an individual with a positive result has the disease (The probability that an individual who tests positive actually has the disease)

Calculation

$$PPV = \frac{\text{diseased with positive test}}{\text{all with positive test}}$$

$$= \frac{\text{True Positives (TP)}}{\text{True Positives (TP)} + \text{False Positives (FP)}}$$

7.2.6 Negative Predictive Value (NPV)

It is the probability that an individual with a negative result does not have the disease T (the probability that an individual who tests negative actually does not have the disease)

Calculation

$$NPV = \frac{\text{disease} - \text{free with negative test}}{\text{all with negative test}}$$

$$= \frac{\text{True Negatives (TN)}}{\text{True Negatives (TN)} + \text{False Negatives (FN)}}$$

7.3 PROBABILITIES AND LIKELIHOOD

7.3.1 Pre-test Probability (Prevalence)

Pre-test probability refers to the likelihood that an individual has a disease within a given population before any testing is performed. Essentially, it reflects the prevalence of the disease in the population.

Calculation

$$\text{pre} - \text{test probability} = \frac{\text{number with disease}}{\text{total number of individuals in study}}$$

7.3.2 Post-test Probabilities

Post-test probability refers to the likelihood that an individual has a disease within a given population after any testing is performed. Positive Predictive Value (PPV) and Negative Predictive Value (NPV) are measures of post-test probabilities, and they are influenced by disease prevalence, which impacts the number of true negatives (TN) and false negatives (FN).

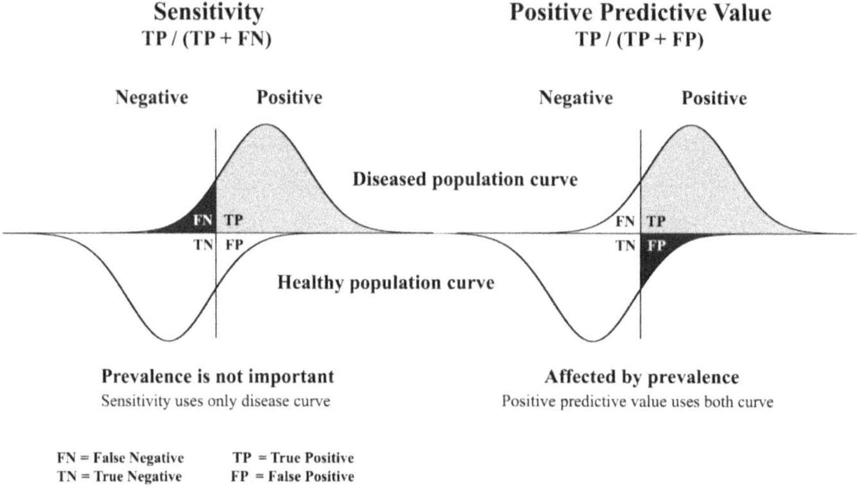

▲ **Figure 7.2:** Effect of prevalence on sensitivity and positive predictive value

For example, in a population with a high disease prevalence (when prevalence is close to 100%), almost all positive results will be true positives (TP), with very few true negatives (TN), and most negative results will be false negatives (FN), with almost no false positives (FP). In this case, the NPV will be close to 0%, while the PPV will approach 100%. As prevalence increases, NPV decreases, and PPV increases.

Conversely, in a population with low disease prevalence (when prevalence is close to 0%), even if the test result is positive, it is most likely to be a false positive (FP) with fewer false negatives (FN). This situation increases NPV and decreases PPV.

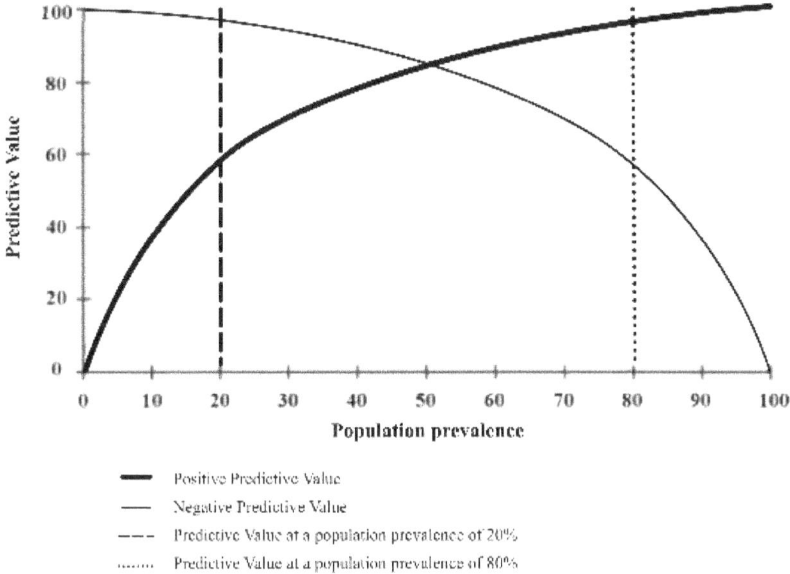

▲ **Figure 7.3:** Effect of prevalence on predictive values

How to remember:
Prevalence and Positive starts with **P**
low **Prevalence** → low **PPV** and high NPV
Disease prevalence has no effect on sensitivity and specificity.

7.3.3   Positive Likelihood Ratio (LR+)

It is the probability of an individual with the disease testing positive divided by the probability of an individual without the disease testing positive

Calculation:

$$LR(+) = \frac{Sensitivity}{1 - Specificity}$$

7.3.4   Negative Likelihood Ratio (LR-)

It is the probability of an individual with the disease testing negative divided by the probability of an individual without the disease testing negative.

Calculation:

$$LR(-) = \frac{1 - Sensitivity}{Specificity}$$

7.4 RECEIVER OPERATING CHARACTERISTIC (ROC) CURVE

The accuracy of screening or diagnostic tests (defined as the number of true positives plus true negatives divided by the number of all observations) is generally quantified by the area under the ROC curve (AUC). ROC (receiver operating characteristic) curves are created by plotting sensitivity (true-positive rate) against 1 – specificity (false-positive rate) for various cutoff thresholds (ie, the value that determines if a given test result is positive or negative). A highly accurate test is highly sensitive (high true-positive rate) and highly specific (low false-positive rate). The more accurate the test is (ie, the higher sensitivity and specificity), the closer the AUC value is to 1.0. Therefore, tests with higher AUCs are more accurate than tests with lower AUCs.

The accuracy of screening or diagnostic tests is quantified by the area under the ROC curve (AUC). The more accurate the test is (ie, higher sensitivity and specificity), the closer the AUC value is to 1.0.

Tests with higher AUCs are more accurate than tests with lower AUCs.

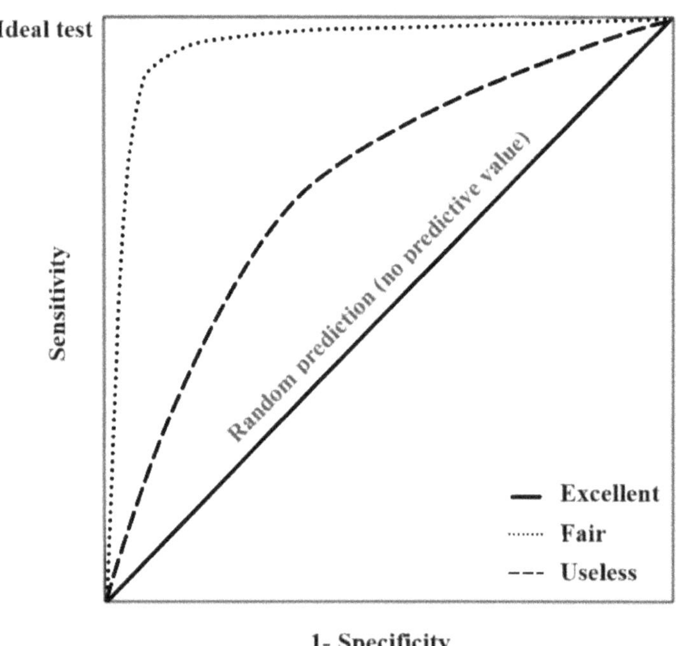

▲ **Figure 7.4:** Interpretation of Area under the ROC curve

7.5   CUTOFF VALUE AND CHANGES IN SENSITIVITY AND SPECIFICITY

The cutoff value of a quantitative diagnostic test determines whether a given result interpreted as positive or negative. Depending on the disease or condition being tested for sensitivity or specificity may be preferred and cutoff value adjusted accordingly. A cutoff value just outside the overlapping region of the curves can maximize the sensitivity or specificity at 100% by correctly classifying all diseased or healthy individual respectively.

When there is overlap between the values of the healthy and diseased populations, a cutoff value that correctly categorizes all individuals in both populations cannot be chosen. This limits the sensitivity and specificity of the test due to the presence of false positive (FP) and/or false negative (FN) individuals. The degree of overlap between the healthy and the diseased population curves limits the maximum combined sensitivity and specificity of a quantitative diagnostic test. The degree to which sensitivity or specificity is affected depends on the chosen cutoff value.

Changing the cutoff point to a lower value (shift to the left) would cause more patients with disease to be test positive (increasing TP, and decrease FN), increasing the sensitivity of the test. However, as a consequence, more patient without disease would also test positive (decreased TN, increase FP), resulting in decreased specificity.

Changing the cutoff point to a higher value (shift to the right) would cause less patients with disease to be test positive (decreasing TP, and increase FN), decreasing the sensitivity of the test. However, as a consequence, less patient without disease would also test positive (increased TN, decrease FP), resulting in increased specificity.

Remember: Low cut-off → more sensitive; (increased TP, and FP)

High cut-off → more specific (increase FN, and TN)

Less overlap → high sensitivity and specificity

7.6   APPLICATIONS

Sensitivity represents the ability of a test to correctly identify those with a given disease. Specificity represents the ability of a test to correctly identify those without a given disease. A good screening tool should be highly sensitive and a test with high specificity are mainly used for confirmatory test.

Cutoff value defines the appropriateness of a test to limit the lead-time bias and length bias. Lowering the cutoff value increases the sensitivity.

Possible Questions from this chapter

- Differentiation of precision and accuracy.
- Calculate false positive and false negative.
- Calculate sensitivity and specificity.
- Identify the use of sensitivity and specificity.
- Calculate Positive predictive value and Negative predictive value.
- Interpret the finding of PPV and NPV.
- Identify the application of PPV and NPV.
- Identify the parameter for diagnostic accuracy.
- Identify the effect of cutoff value on sensitivity.

Questions on Precision and Accuracy

79. A laboratory technician is testing a new glucose meter. The meter is used to test the blood glucose level of a patient three times, resulting in readings of 85 mg/dL, 88 mg/dL, and 90 mg/dL. While the readings are consistent, the true glucose level, as determined by a standard laboratory test, is actually 100 mg/dL. Which of the following parameters is most likely to be low based on these glucose meter results?

    A. Accuracy
    B. Precision
    C. Sensitivity
    D. Specificity
    E. Validity

    Answer A: Accuracy. Repeated measurements provide similar results, but they are not close to the actual blood pressure values. Therefore, this glucose meter has low accuracy.

80. A 45-year-old woman visits the clinic for a routine check-up. During her visit, her blood pressure is measured three times using the same device, yielding readings of 120/80 mmHg, 135/88 mmHg, and 115/68 mmHg Which of the following parameters is most likely to be low based on the results of these blood pressure measurements?

A. Accuracy

B. Precision

C. Sensitivity

D. Specificity

E. Validity

Answer B: Precision. Repeated measurements provide diverse results. Therefore, this sphygmomanometer is low precision.

Questions on Calculation of False Positive and False Negative

81. A new rapid test for detecting COVID-19 is being evaluated against ELISA, which is considered the gold standard. In a study of 700 patients, 100 are found to have COVID-19 infection by ELISA. The rapid test shows a sensitivity of 85% and a specificity of 95%. How many false positives are present in the study?

A. 5

B. 15

C. 30

D. 100

E. 600

Answer: C. 30. With a specificity of 95%, the false positive rate is 5%. Applying this to 600 non-diseased individuals (700 total - 100 diseased), 5% of 600 is 30, meaning there are 30 false positives.

(Remember: To calculate false **P**ositive – use s**P**ecificity)

82. A research team is investigating urinary my prostate score (MPS2) for diagnosing prostate cancer. They recruit 100 patients who are known to have prostate cancer and 300 patients who do not have the disease. The results show that the test has a sensitivity of 85% and a specificity of 75%. Based on this data, which of the following is the approximate number of false negative results in this study?

A. 15

B. 25

C. 30

D. 45

E. 50

Answer A.15. With a sensitivity of 85%, the false negative rate is 15%. Applying this to 100 diseased individuals, 15% of 100 is 15, meaning there are 15 false negatives.
(Remember: To calculate false **N**egative – use se**N**sitivity)

Questions on Calculation of Sensitivity and Specificity

83. The results of a study evaluating a new diagnostic test for detecting pneumonia are shown in the table below.

	Pneumonia	No Pneumonia
Test positive	120	40
Test negative	30	210

What is the sensitivity of the new diagnostic test?

A. 16%

B. 25%

C. 75%

D. 80%

E. 84%

F. 87.5%

Answer: D. 80%. Sensitivity refers to the proportion of true positive cases detected by the test among all individuals with the disease.

$$\text{Sensitivity} = \frac{\text{True Positives}}{\text{All Diseased Individuals}} = \frac{120}{(120+30)} = \frac{120}{150} = 80\%$$

84. A new diagnostic test for identifying celiac disease is under evaluation. The comparison gold standard is a positive blood test plus biopsy. The results of the study are given below:

	celiac disease present	celiac disease absent
Test positive	80	20
Test negative	120	180

What is the specificity of the new test?

A. 10%

B. 40%

C. 60%

D. 80%

E. 90%

Answer: E. 90%. Specificity refers to the proportion of true negative cases detected by the test among all individuals without the disease.

$$\text{Specificity} = \frac{\text{True Negative}}{\text{All Non Diseased Individuals}} = \frac{180}{(180+20)} = \frac{180}{200} = 90\%$$

85. A study is conducted to assess whether the detection of Phosphorylated tau (p-tau) 217 immunoassay, in blood can improve the diagnosis of Alzheimer's disease. A total of 500 individuals (200 Alzheimer's patients and 300 healthy controls) are tested. The results show that 160 of the Alzheimer's patients have a high level of p-tau 217, while 20 of the healthy controls also have a high level of p-tau 217. A high level of p-tau 217is considered a positive test for Alzheimer's disease. Which of the following values best represents the specificity of this test?

A. 7%

B. 50%

C. 67%

D. 80%

E. 93%

Answer: E. 93%. Based on the information, 280 of healthy will be truly negative with low level of p-tau 217. Specificity refers to the proportion of true negative cases detected by the test among all individuals without the disease.

$$\text{Specificity} = \frac{\text{True Negative}}{\text{All Non Diseased Individuals}} = \frac{280}{320} = 93\%$$

Questions on application and interpretation of sensitivity and specificity

86. Galactosemia is an inherited disorder where the body cannot properly process galactose, a sugar found in milk. If untreated, affected infants can suffer from liver damage, cataracts, intellectual disability, and even death. Galactosemia is screened for in newborns to prevent these severe outcomes. The estimated incidence is about 1 in 60,000 newborns. If all newborns are tested, the goal should be to identify as many true cases as possible in order to prevent irreversible damage. Therefore, this screening test should be designed to have a high:

    A. Negative predictive value

    B. Number of false positives

    C. Positive predictive value

    D. Sensitivity

    E. Specificity

    Answer: D. Sensitivity. While an ideal screening test would possess both high sensitivity and specificity, achieving both characteristics is often challenging. In screening for life-threatening diseases, it is crucial to identify all individuals who may have these conditions. A highly sensitive test ensures that most patients with the disease receive positive results, resulting in fewer false negatives and minimizing the number of missed cases.

    NB: A highly sensitive test identifies most patients with the disease, minimizing false negatives, making a negative result useful for ruling out the condition ("SnNout"). A highly specific test reduces false positives, making a positive result reliable for confirming the disease ("SpPin").

87. The specificity of the current test for detecting disease Y in the general population is 80%. A group of scientists aims to develop a new test that improves specificity for detecting disease Y. They conduct a study on a random sample from the general population. The study results are shown below:

	Patients with disease	Patients without disease
Test positive	320	60
Test negative	40	340

According to these results, have the researchers achieved their goal?

A. Cannot be determined because the prevalence of disease Y is not provided

B. No, the new test has about 10% lower specificity than the standard test

C. No, the researchers' test leads to nearly the same specificity as the standard test

D. Yes, the researchers achieved an increase in specificity of about 5%

E. Yes, the researchers achieved an increase in specificity of about 8%

Answer: D. Yes, the researchers achieved an increase in specificity of about 5%. Existing specificity is 80%. The new specificity is calculated as: Specificity = 340/400 = 85%. This represents a 5% increase compared to the previous specificity.

88. A study evaluates the performance of carbohydrate antigen 19-9 (CA19-9) as a new serum marker for the early detection of pancreatic cancer among at-risk individuals. The analysis reveals that a marker value ≥ 100.0 U/mL has a sensitivity of 68% and a specificity of 98% for predicting pancreatic cancer. Which of the following conclusions about the study results is correct?

A. Based on a cut point of ≥ 100.0 U/mL, 2% of individuals without pancreatic cancer will be incorrectly identified.

B. Based on a cut point of ≥ 100.0 U/mL, 32% of individuals with pancreatic cancer will be correctly identified.

C. Based on a cut point of ≥ 100.0 U/mL, 68% of individuals with pancreatic cancer will be incorrectly identified.

D. Based on a cut point of ≥ 100.0 U/mL, 98% of individuals with pancreatic cancer will be correctly identified.

E. Based on a cut point of ≥ 100.0 U/mL, 98% of individuals without pancreatic cancer will be incorrectly identified.

Answer. A. Based on a cut point of ≥ 100.0 U/mL, 2% of individuals without pancreatic cancer will be incorrectly identified. The specificity of this test is 98%, 98% means those without pancreatic cancer will correctly identify as non-cancer, where as 2% of the non-cancer patients will incorrectly identify as cancer patient.

Questions on calculation of PPV and NPV

89. A 45-year-old woman with a history of diabetes and smoking presents to the clinic with shortness of breath and fatigue. A coronary calcium scan was performed to assess for coronary atherosclerosis. A recent study comparing the coronary calcium scan to cardiac catheterization, the gold standard for diagnosing coronary atherosclerosis, yielded the following results:

coronary calcium scan	coronary atherosclerosis present	coronary atherosclerosis absent
Test positive	160	40
Test negative	140	260

The patient tests positive on coronary calcium scan. Assuming her pre-test probability is equivalent to the prevalence of coronary atherosclerosis in the study, what is the probability that the patient has CHF?

    A.   53%

    B.   65%

    C.   70%

    D.   80%

    E.   86%

Answer: D. 80%. $\text{PPV} = \dfrac{\text{True Positive}}{\text{All with Positve test}} = \dfrac{160}{(160+40)} = 80\%$

90. A general practitioner evaluates a population of 1,000 adults using a new test to diagnose diabetes. The prevalence of diabetes in the population is 10%. The sensitivity of the diagnostic test is 90% and the specificity is 80%. Which of the following is the likelihood that an adult with a positive test result truly has diabetes?

    A.   10 / (10+720)

    B.   90 / (90+180)

    C.   90 / (90+200)

    D.   180 / (180+720)

    E.   720 / (720+10)

Answer: B. 90 / (90+180). The prevalence is 10%, meaning there are 100 individuals with diabetes and 900 without. With a sensitivity of 90%, 90 out of 100 individuals with diabetes will test positive. With a specificity of 80%, 20% of the 900 non-diabetic individuals, or 180, will be false positives. Therefore, the total number of positive test results is 90+180=270. Among these, 90 are true positives. Thus, the positive predictive value (PPV) is: 90 / (90+180)

91. Researchers have proposed using low-frequency electromagnetic waves as a screening test for early-stage breast cancer. The initial evaluation of the test reveals the following:

Test finding	Breast Cancer		Total
	Present	Not Present	
Test Positive	65	25	90
Test Negative	10	100	110
Total	75	125	200

Which of the following is the likelihood that a patient with a negative test does not have breast cancer?

A. 0.72

B. 0.80

C. 0.86

D. 0.91

E. 0.97

Answer: D. 0.91. Negative predictive value =

$$\frac{\text{True Negative}}{\text{All with Negative test}} = \frac{100}{(10+100)} = 0.91$$

92. A 72-year-old woman is brought to the hospital with a history of recurrent falls. The attending physician suspects that she may have Parkinson's disease (PD) and uses protein dopa decarboxylase (DCC) as a diagnostic test to help rule it out. Her test result comes back negative. A study evaluating DCC test in a sample of 400 individuals aged ≥70, where the prevalence of Parkinson's disease is 25%, has shown the test to have a specificity of 90% and a sensitivity of 80%. Assuming this patient's pretest probability of having Parkinson's disease is equivalent to the disease prevalence in the study population, what is the probability that this patient truly does not have Parkinson's disease?

    A. 80 / (80+20)

    B. 80 / (80+30)

    C. 270 / (270+20)

    D. 270 / (270+30)

    E. 270 / 400

    Answer: C. 270 / (270+20). The prevalence is 25%, meaning there are 100 individuals with Parkinson's disease and 300 without. With a specificity of 90%, 270 out of 300 individuals without Parkinson's disease will be truly negative. With a sensitivity of 80%, 20% of the 100 Parkin's disease, or 20, will be false negatives. Therefore, the total number of negative test results is 20+270=290. Among these, 270 are true negatives. Thus, the negative predictive value (NPV) is: 270 / (270+20).

Questions on interpretation of PPV and NPV findings

93. A researcher uses carbohydrate antigen 19-9 (CA19-9) to detect early-stage pancreatic cancer. The test has a sensitivity of 81% and a specificity of 90% at cut off point of 37 U/mL when compared to CT scan and biopsy. The test is applied in two different populations: a low-risk population in Canada, where 10 out of 100,000 people have pancreatic cancer, and a high-risk population in India, where 150 out of 100,000 people are diagnosed with pancreatic cancer. Which of the following is the most accurate statement about this test?

    A. Negative predictive value of the test is lower in the Indian population

    B. Positive predictive value of the test is higher in the Canadian population

C. Sensitivity of the test is higher in the Canadian population

D. Specificity of the test is higher in the Indian population

E. The test is not reliable in the Canadian population

Answer: A. Negative predictive value of the test is lower in the Indian population. Sensitivity and specificity are not influenced by disease prevalence, but positive and negative predictive values are. A higher disease prevalence increases the PPV but decreases the NPV.

94. A new blood test is developed to diagnose small cell adenocarcinoma in a population of 1,200 men age ≥ 50. The test has a sensitivity of 85% and a specificity of 92%. The test is then used in 2 other populations of men of the same age: population 1 has a prevalence of lung cancer of 10%, and population 2 has a prevalence of 25%. Which of the following best describes how the negative predictive values (NPV) and the positive predictive values (PPV) from populations 1 and 2 relate to each other?

    A. NPV and PPV do not change as prevalence changes

    B. NPV in population 1 < NPV population 2; PPV in population 1 < PPV population 2

    C. NPV in population 1 < NPV population 2; PPV in population 1 > PPV population 2

    D. NPV in population 1 > NPV population 2; PPV in population 1 < PPV population 2

    E. NPV in population 1 > NPV population 2; PPV in population 1 > PPV population 2

Answer: D. NPV in population 1 > NPV population 2; PPV in population 1 < PPV population 2. Positive and negative predictive values are not influenced by disease prevalence. A higher disease prevalence increases the PPV but decreases the NPV. Population 2 has higher prevalences, thus it would have lower negative predictive value and higher positive predictive value than population 1.

Questions on the application of PPV and NPV

95. A new rapid diagnostic test for tuberculosis is being developed. The test is designed to detect TB antigens in the blood. Two populations with differing TB prevalence levels are selected to evaluate the test's performance. The researchers aim to compare the diagnostic accuracy of the test across both populations. Which of the following test parameters is most likely to differ between the two populations?

A. Negative likelihood ratio

B. Positive likelihood ratio

C. Positive predictive value

D. Sensitivity

E. Specificity

Answer: C. Positive predictive value. Predictive values are performance measures of a diagnostic test that vary with the prevalence of the disease in the population of interest.

96. A 30-year-old man comes to the office after undergoing a screening test for hepatitis C virus (HCV) due to a history of intravenous drug use. The results of his HCV antibody test come back negative. He asks, "What are the chances that I really do not have hepatitis C?" Which of the following diagnostic test parameters would be most useful for answering this patient's question?

A. Negative predictive value

B. Positive predictive value

C. Reliability

D. Sensitivity

E. Specificity

Answer: A. Negative predictive value. Negative predictive value (NPV) refers to the likelihood that a person does not have a disease when their test result is negative. It is determined by dividing the number of true negative results by the total number of negative tests (both true and false negatives). NPV is influenced by the prevalence of the disease within the target population.

The prevalence of a disease can serves as an estimate for the pretest probability of a patient having the condition, especially if the patient closely resembles the population. When a patient has a high pretest probability, the NPV of a negative test result will be lower. Conversely, a patient with a low pretest probability will have a higher NPV with a negative result.

In this case, the patient's pretest probability of having hepatitis C is elevated, likely due to history of intravenous drug use. As a result, his negative HCV antibody test would have a lower NPV compared to another patient without any hepatitis C risk factors who also receives a negative result.

Questions on factors determining diagnostic accuracy

97. A clinical study investigates the ability of 5 different cutoff values of plasma thrombin–antithrombin complex (TAT) to predict stroke severity and outcome of acute ischemic stroke. Researchers assess the sensitivity, specificity, and area under the curve (AUC) for each blood plasma TAT level:

Cut-off value	Sensitivity (%)	Specificity (%)	AUC
Value 1	50.0	80.0	0.650
Value 2	72.5	75.0	0.780
Value 3	83.3	85.0	0.890
Value 4	65.0	60.0	0.720
Value 5	90.0	65.0	0.800

Which blood cutoff value is most accurate?
A. 1
B. 2
C. 3
D. 4
E. 5

Answer: C. 3. The accuracy of screening or diagnostic tests is quantified by the area under the ROC curve (AUC). The more accurate the test is (ie, higher sensitivity and specificity), the closer the AUC value is to 1.0. Tests with higher AUCs are more accurate than tests with lower AUCs. In this case, Cut-off value 3, provides the highest AUC, is the most accurate value.

Questions on effect of change in cutoff value on sensitivity and specificity

98. Carbohydrate antigen 19-9 (CA19-9) is being assessed for its effectiveness in detecting early-stage pancreatic cancer. Elevated CA19-9 levels (measured in U/mL) have been observed in patients with confirmed pancreatic cancer. A study included 250 healthy volunteers and 220 patients with biopsy-confirmed lung cancer, and their CA19-9 levels were represented in a graph. The researchers determined the sensitivity and specificity of CA19-9 using a cutoff of 37 U/mL (solid vertical line). If they had chosen a higher cutoff, indicated by a dashed line at 100 U/mL, what impact would this change most likely have?

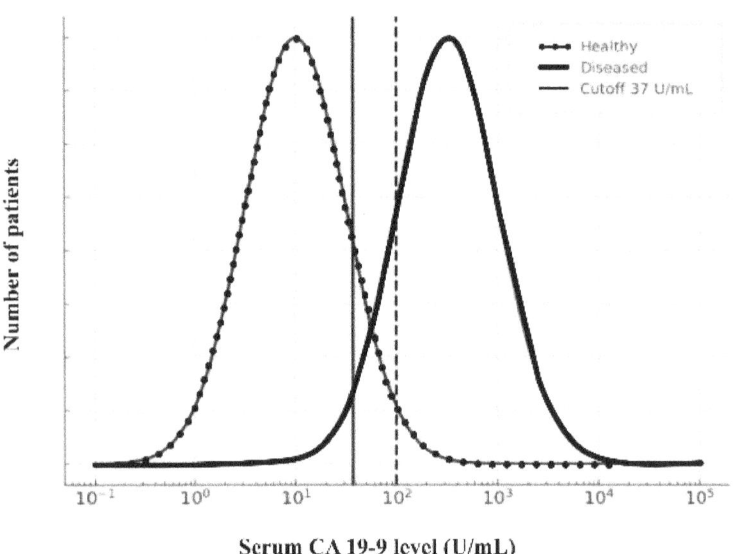

Serum CA 19-9 level (U/mL)

A. Higher sensitivity

B. Higher number of false positives

C. Lower number of true negatives

D. Lower sensitivity

E. Higher number of true positives

Answer: D. Lower sensitivity. When the cutoff value is increase from 37 U/mL to 100 U/mL, the test becomes less capable of detecting cases of the disease, thereby decreasing its sensitivity.

99. A new blood marker is being investigated for its potential to diagnose early-stage prostate cancer. A sample of 500 men is divided into two groups based on the presence or absence of a family history of prostate cancer. Blood levels of the new marker are obtained for both groups, and conventional diagnostic testing is used to determine their disease status. The graph on the top represents the distribution of the marker in men with a family history, and the graph on the bottom represents the distribution in men without a family history.

Family History Present

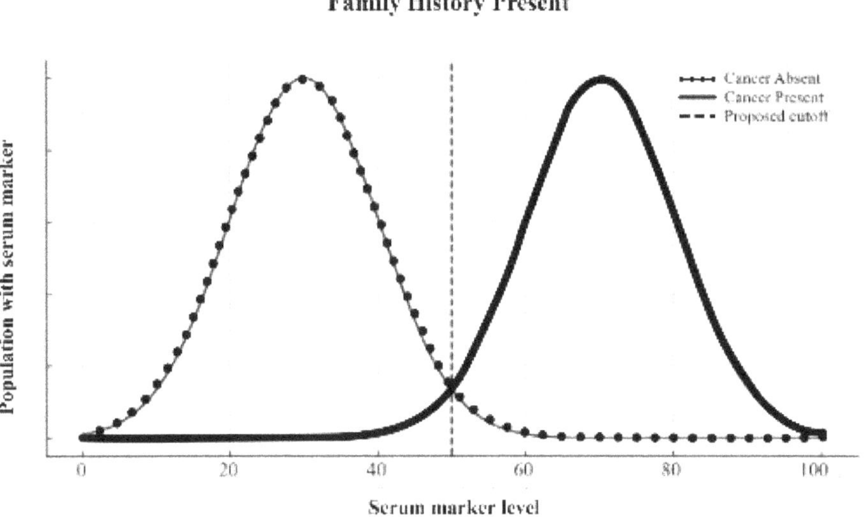

Family History Absent

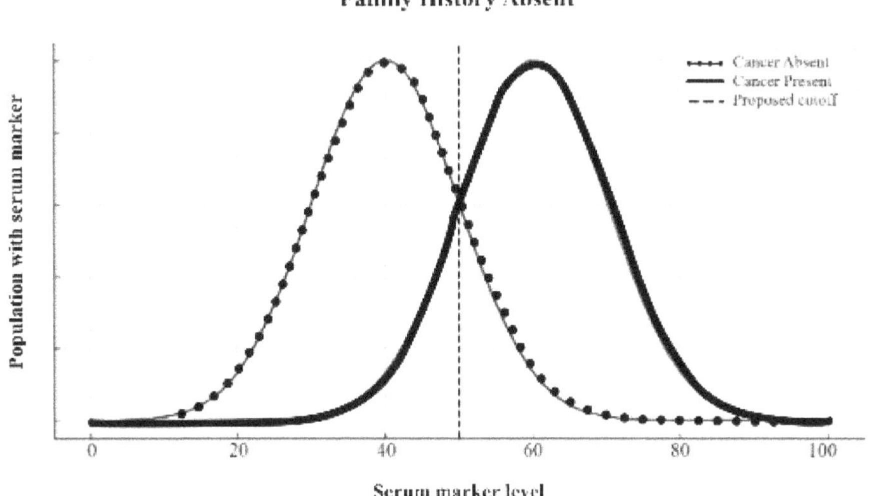

The proposed cutoff value for the blood marker is shown. Use of the new marker in men with a family history of prostate cancer, compared with those without a family history, is associated with which of the following?

A. Higher sensitivity and higher specificity

B. Higher sensitivity and lower specificity

C. Higher sensitivity and same specificity

D. Lower sensitivity and higher specificity

E. Lower sensitivity and lower specificity

F. Lower sensitivity and unchanged specificity

G. Unchanged sensitivity and unchanged specificity

Answer: A. Higher sensitivity and higher specificity. The cutoff value in a quantitative diagnostic test determines whether a result is classified as positive or negative. If there is overlap between the serum values of healthy and diseased individuals, it becomes impossible to select a cutoff that perfectly distinguishes between the two groups. As a result, the test's sensitivity and specificity are reduced due to the occurrence of false positives (FPs) and false negatives (FNs).

Sensitivity refers to how well a test identifies individuals with the disease, calculated by dividing the number of true positives (TP) by the total number of people with the disease (TP / [TP + FN]). **Sensitivity** $= \dfrac{\text{TP}}{\text{TP} + \textbf{FN}}$. Specificity measures the test's ability to correctly identify individuals without the disease, calculated as the number of true negatives (TN) divided by the total number of individuals without the disease (TN / [TN + FP]). **Specificity** $= = \dfrac{\text{TN}}{\text{TN} + \textbf{FP}}$.

In this example, the serum marker in women with **Family history** shows **less overlap** between healthy and diseased groups (seen in the upper curves) compared to those without family history (represented by the lower curves). This reduction in overlap decreases the number of FPs and FNs, resulting in a serum marker with **greater sensitivity and specificity** (i.e., improved accuracy) in women with Family history.

Family History Present

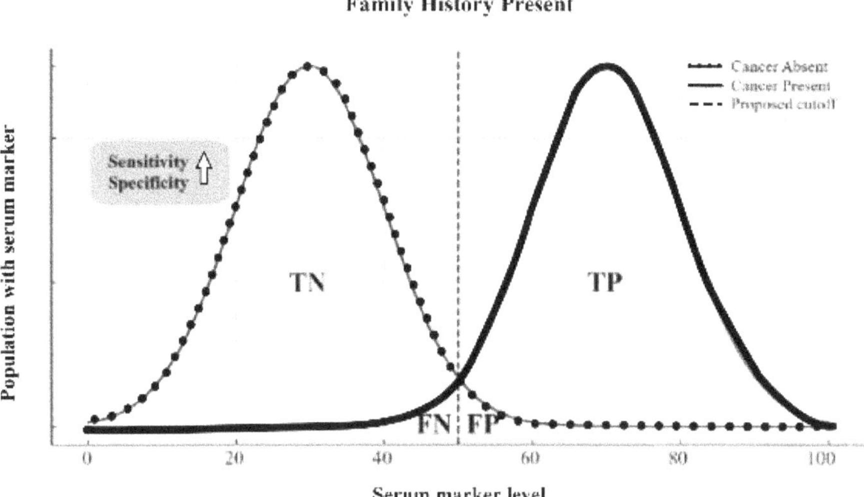

Family History Absent

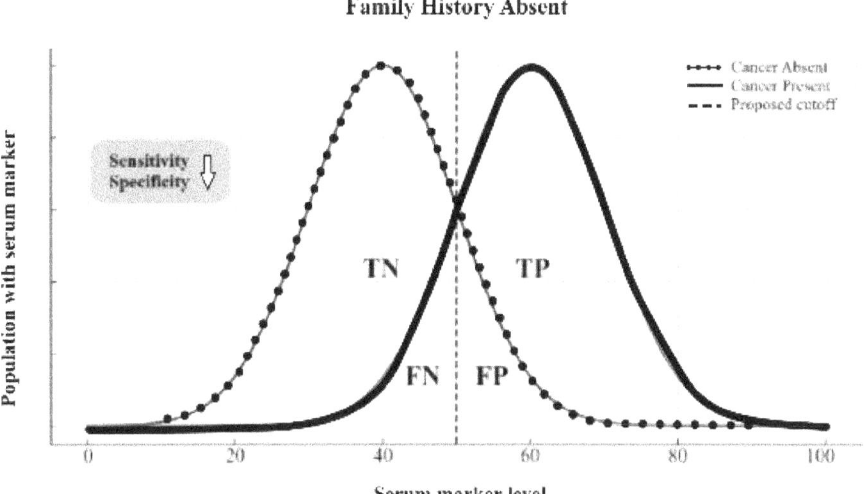

08   BIAS AND ERRORS

In this chapter, we discuss common types of biases and sources of errors arising from study design or data analysis, as well as strategies to overcome these issues.

LEARNING OUTCOME:

1. Identify the causes of error and different types of bias.
2. List the situation susceptible to each bias.
3. Propose an appropriate approach to minimize these bias.

Understanding biases and errors is critical when conducting or interpreting research, as they can significantly affect the validity of results.

8.1   ERROR

Error refers to the difference between the predicted values in a study and the actual true values.

Beta Error (Type II Error)

When a study fails to reject a false null hypothesis, meaning it fails to detect a real effect, and is known as beta (Type II error). This often happens when a study has a small sample size, resulting in insufficient statistical power and leading to a false negative result.

8.2   BIAS

Bias refers to a systematic deviation from the truth during data collection, analysis, or interpretation, resulting in an overestimation or underestimation of the effect of a drug, intervention, or exposure.

8.2.1 Selection Bias

Selection bias is a type of error that occurs when sample that does not represent the general population, mainly due to non-random sample selection.

A) Volunteer Bias and Non-response Bias

Volunteers may differ from the general (target) population, and non-responders often have different characteristics from responders.

Patients with cancer who do not respond to standard treatments are more likely to join experimental trials (self-selection). This can result in findings that don't apply to patients with less advanced cancers. (volunteer bias)

In a mental health survey, people with severe depression may be less likely to respond, leading to skewed results (non-response bias). This type of bias is common in studies using mailed surveys or questionnaires

B) Healthy Worker Bias

When comparing workers to the general population, workers appear healthier simply because they are fit to work.

A study compares the health outcomes of factory workers to the general population, leading to overestimation of health in workers group. (healthy worker bias)

C) Berkson's Bias

In case-control studies using hospital controls, where controls are hospitalized due to an exposure which is also related to the outcome factor being studied, weakening the effect measure, i.e. biased toward the null hypothesis of no association.

In a case-control study on diabetes and heart disease, researchers use hospitalized patients as controls. Since hospitalized patients often have other conditions like diabetes, this can underestimate the link between diabetes and heart disease, as both groups have a higher prevalence of diabetes than the general population. (Berkson's bias)

D) Referral (Admission Rate) Bias

When certain populations are more likely to be referred to specialized care, the association between exposure and outcome are exaggerated.

In a study on asbestos and lung cancer at a hospital specializing in asbestosis, lung cancer patients may have had more asbestos exposure than the general population, leading to an overestimation of the link between asbestos and lung cancer. (Referral/Admission bias)

E) Allocation Bias

In clinical trials, when subjects are non-randomly assigned to treatment groups, the results may be skewed in either direction, depending on the differences between the groups.

If sicker patients are more likely to be placed in the treatment group, it may exaggerate the treatment effect if the treatment is effective. Conversely, if healthier patients are allocated to the control group, it might lead to an underestimation of the treatment's effectiveness (bias towards the null).

F) Attrition Bias

Attrition bias, a type of selection bias, can occur due to unequal loss to follow-up between study groups. Lost subjects may differ in their risk of developing the outcome compared to those who remain. Attrition bias is less likely if losses are random across groups, as this only reduces the study population.

Withdrawal bias, a subset of attrition bias, occurs when participants with undesirable outcomes or those lost to follow-up are excluded from the study.

Intention-to-treat (ITT) analysis helps mitigate bias by including all participants and accounting for cross-overs and attrition.

8.2.2 Misclassification Bias

Bias may be introduced when subjects are incorrectly classified with regard to their exposure status, outcome status or both.

Nondifferential misclassification occurs when misclassification rates are equal between groups, making them appear more similar than they actually are. This pushes the association toward the null value (e.g., an odds ratio of 1), leading to a bias toward the null hypothesis.

Differential misclassification, on the other hand, occurs when misclassification rates differ between groups, which can shift the association either toward or away from the null value.

A) Measurement Bias

A systematic error in measuring outcomes or exposures

When a faulty sphygmomanometer is used, there is a risk of misclassifying individuals into hypertensive or normotensive groups.

B) Recall Bias

When participants inaccurately recall past exposures, their exposure status may be misclassified. This type of bias is common in case-control studies.

In a lung cancer study, patients with cancer may better remember their smoking history, while healthy participants might forget or underreport. (recall bias).

C) Detection Bias

When outcomes are detected differently between groups, such as more frequent testing in one group, the finding is likely to be biased.

Subjects may undergo more frequent surveillance due to having a risk factor or being exposed to the study intervention, which would detect more diseases compared to those who are not.

D) Observer Bias

When a researcher's expectations or beliefs unconsciously influence how they perceive or record data, particularly in subjective outcomes (such as interpreting clinical signs or imaging results), inaccurate finding may occur.

A researcher knows which patients received a new treatment versus a placebo, they may unintentionally interpret results in favour of the treatment, leading to inaccurate findings. (observer bias). Double-blind studies, where both participants and researchers are unaware of treatment assignments, or using independent observers to verify data, can reduce this bias.

8.2.3 Psychological Biases

Poorly blinded studies can influence how participants and researchers perceive, interpret, and respond to information, potentially distorting judgment and leading to biased outcomes.

A) Hawthorne Effect

Participants may change their behaviour simply because they are aware of being observed, which can affect the study's results and potentially compromise its validity. This is common in studies involving behavioural outcomes.

A study on the components of physicians' history-taking found that they may take a more thorough medical history when aware that their behaviour is being monitored. (Hawthorne effect)

B) Pygmalion (Rosenthal) Effect

Researchers' expectations can influence participants' performance, resulting in a self-fulfilling prophecy.

In a nursing home setting, nurses who are told that certain patients will progress more quickly in rehabilitation may unintentionally provide those patients with more attention, resulting in better outcomes compared to those with average expectations. (Pygmalion effect)

C) Placebo Effect

An improvement in a patient's condition that occurs due to their belief in the treatment, rather than the treatment itself.

A patient reports reduced pain after taking a placebo, believing it to be a powerful medication.

D) Ascertainment Bias

Clinical trial results are distorted when participants or researchers know which intervention each participant is receiving, influencing the results.

If a participant knows they are receiving a placebo, they may be less likely to report benefits related to the placebo effect. As a result, the comparison between the treatment and control groups is distorted.

NB:

In some contexts, ascertainment bias also refers to selection bias that occurs when certain groups or individuals are more likely to be identified, observed, or selected for a study due to the methods used. This leads to skewed or unrepresentative findings.

In a medical study, patients with more severe symptoms may be more likely to be diagnosed and included, while those with mild or no symptoms may be overlooked, leading to an overestimation of the condition's severity.

8.2.4 Biases Related to Timing

Inaccurate conclusions about the relationship between an intervention and the outcome can also arise from the timing of an intervention or measurement.

A) Lead-time Bias

A screening test detects a disease earlier than a clinical diagnosis, falsely suggesting longer survival without actually changing the prognosis.

A 55-year-old woman undergoes a routine cancer screening and is diagnosed with early-stage cancer. Her friend, who didn't get screened, is diagnosed with the same cancer two years later when symptoms appear. Both women live until age 65, but the screened woman appears to have survived longer with the disease, even though the outcome and prognosis were the same.

B) Length-time Bias

Screening tends to detect slower-progressing diseases, which overestimates the benefits of screening.

A new blood test is developed for detecting a type of leukaemia. The test mainly identifies cases with slower progression. Tom, who gets tested, is diagnosed with this slow-progressing leukaemia. His colleague, Sara, who only gets diagnosed when symptoms become severe, has a faster-progressing form of the disease. Tom's condition appears to have a better prognosis due to early detection, but in reality, the survival rates for both types of leukaemia are similar.

8.2.5 Misinterpretation of Data

Ecological Fallacy

An association observed at the population level is incorrectly applied to individuals.

A study finds that countries with higher average income have lower rates of heart disease. It might be incorrectly assumed that individuals with higher income within a country also have lower rates of heart disease.

8.3 OTHER SOURCES OF BIAS

Certain factors may lead to bias if they are not properly addressed/ managed.

8.3.1 Confounding

When a third variable (a confounder) is associated with both the exposure and the outcome, their relationship may be distorted.

Fatty food intake could be a confounder in a study evaluating the association between physical activity and obesity, as people who do not exercise regularly may be more likely to consume a high-fat diet.

Techniques like matching, stratification, and randomization help reduce confounding.

8.3.2 Accumulation Effect

Prolonged or repeated exposure to a risk factor can gradually influence outcomes. The impact of this exposure depends on both its duration and intensity. Often, long-term exposure is needed before the effect on the disease process becomes clinically apparent. Studies that overlook the increased risk associated with longer exposure may underestimate the link between exposure and disease.

8.3.3 Latent Period

The latent period refers to the time between exposure to a risk factor and the onset of detectable disease. While the latent period itself is not a bias, failing to account for it properly can lead to biases such as lead-time bias.

8.4 A NATURAL PHENOMENON OFTEN MISTAKEN FOR BIAS

8.4.1 Effect Modification

Effect modification occurs when the effect of an exposure on an outcome is modified by another variable. It is often mistaken for confounding, but stratified analysis—dividing the cohort into subgroups—can differentiate between the two. In cases of effect modification, the various strata will show different measures of association, whereas with confounding, stratification typically reveals no significant differences between the groups.

Effect modification is not a bias, as it does not arise from design flaws or analytical errors in the study. Instead, it is a natural phenomenon that should be acknowledged and described rather than corrected.

Possible questions from this chapter

- Identify type of error/bias affecting the validity of study finding
- Identify the approaches to minimize the error/bias

Questions on identification of factors / types of bias affecting the validity of study finding

100. A researcher is conducting a randomized controlled trial to evaluate the effect of a new dietary intervention on reducing blood pressure in hypertensive patients. The study involves 40 participants, randomly assigned to either the intervention or a standard diet group (20 patients in each group). After 3 months, the reduction in blood pressure is 10 mmHg in the intervention group and 5 mmHg in the standard diet group, but the difference is not statistically significant ($p = 0.25$). The researcher concludes that the new dietary intervention does not reduce blood pressure. Which of the following is most likely to explain these results?

   A. Ascertainment bias

   B. Effect modification

   C. Insufficient statistical power

   D. Recall bias

   E. Selection bias

   Answer: C. Insufficient statistical power. When the sample size is small, the findings may not be statistically significant due to insufficient statistical power.

101. A clinical trial is conducted to evaluate the effect of a new cholesterol-lowering drug on the risk of cardiovascular events. The study reports a relative risk (RR) of 0.85 ($p = 0.08$) for cardiovascular events in the drug group compared to the placebo group. Based on a significance level of $\alpha = 0.05$, the researchers conclude that the drug does not significantly reduce cardiovascular risk. However, a later meta-analysis finds a significant reduction in cardiovascular events with the drug ($RR = 0.82$, $p = 0.02$). What is the most likely issue with the original study?

   A. Lead-time bias

   B. Observer bias

   C. Poor randomization

   D. Sample size

   E. Selection bias

Answer: D. Sample size. The first study and the meta-analysis (which combines the results of several studies) reported similar relative risk (RR) outcomes, but they reached different conclusions. The meta-analysis achieved statistical significance ($p < \alpha = 0.05$), whereas the first study did not. The most likely reason for this discrepancy is that the larger meta-analysis more accurately reflects the true effect of the cholesterol-lowering drug in reducing cardiovascular risk. In contrast, the first study likely made a Type II (β) error, falsely concluding that there was no reduction in cardiovascular risk.

A Type II error occurs when a study fails to detect a difference that actually exists, and this error is related to the study's statistical power (power = 1 - β). Sample size and power are directly related—studies with larger sample sizes have greater power to detect differences if they exist. The smaller sample size of the first study meant it was underpowered, making it less likely to detect a difference in outcomes between those who took the new cholesterol-lowering drug and those who did not.

102. A cohort study is designed to examine the link between high-fat diets and the risk of colorectal cancer. Researchers recruit 5000 participants by sending out invitations through social media platforms. Dietary habits are assessed via online questionnaires, and cancer incidence is followed for 10 years. By the end of the study, 1200 participants who had reported high-fat diets at baseline had dropped out. The researchers report no significant association between high-fat diets and colorectal cancer (relative risk = 1.10; 95% CI = 0.85-1.45). What bias is most likely affecting the results?

    A. Confounding

    B. Lead-time bias

    C. Observer bias

    D. Recall bias

    E. Selection bias

Answer: E. Selection bias. Attrition bias, a type of selection bias, can occur when there is unequal loss to follow-up between study groups. Participants who drop out may differ in their risk of developing the outcome compared to those who remain in the study. Attrition bias is less likely if the losses are random across groups, as this would only reduce the study population size. In this study, 1,200 participants from the high-fat diet group dropped out at baseline, making selection bias highly likely.

103. A case-control study is conducted to assess the relationship between cured meat consumption and the risk of pancreatic cancer. Controls are matched to cases based on age and gender. Alcohol consumption is determined through self-reported surveys completed by the participants. On analysis, the odds ratio is 4.2 (95% confidence interval: 1.5-8.0). Which of the following is most likely to affect the validity of this study?

   A. Confounding bias by gender

   B. Measurement error

   C. Misclassification bias

   D. Observer bias

   E. Selection bias

   Answer: C. Misclassification bias. Misclassification bias occurs when subjects are incorrectly categorized with respect to their exposure status, outcome status, or both. In this study, responses rely on questionnaires or interviews to determine exposure status, making it particularly susceptible to misclassification, often in the form of recall bias. For instance, individuals with pancreatic cancer are more likely to report higher meat consumption, leading to differential misclassification.

104. A researcher is investigating the possible link between pesticide exposure and childhood asthma. Parents of children with asthma and parents of children without asthma are asked about their use of pesticides in the home during their child's early years. The study finds that parents of children with asthma are more likely to report frequent pesticide use compared to parents of children without asthma. This study design is most vulnerable to which type of bias?

   A. Allocation bias

   B. Detection bias

   C. Recall bias

   D. Reporting bias

   E. Selection bias

   Answer. C. Recall bias. Recall bias occurs when study participants inaccurately remember past exposures, and it is common in retrospective studies such as case-control studies. Individuals who experience an adverse event are more likely to remember or overestimate potential risk factors compared to those who have not experienced the event. In this case, parents of children with asthma are more likely to report pesticide exposure than parents of healthy children, leading to recall bias.

105. A study is conducted to assess the effectiveness of a new pain management protocol for patients recovering from knee surgery. Nurses who implement the protocol also evaluate the patients' pain levels. It is found that nurses who are involved in the new protocol report significantly lower pain scores than those who are not involved. What is the most likely explanation for this discrepancy?

 A. Confounding
 B. Measurement error
 C. Observer bias
 D. Recall bias
 E. Selection bias

Answer: C. Observer bias. Observer bias occurs when investigators misclassify data due to preconceived expectations or prior knowledge about the study or its participants. This type of bias is especially relevant when outcomes are subjective. In this case, nurses involved in the new protocol may be aware of which patients received the new pain management treatment, potentially leading them to assess pain scores differently.

106. A study is conducted to evaluate the effects of Orlistat, a dietary supplement that inhibits lipase and is used for weight loss. Participants are randomly assigned to either receive the supplement or a placebo. Both the participants and the researchers assessing the results are unaware of who is taking the supplement. The study is designed in such a way to minimize potential bias. What type of bias is this setup most effective at preventing?

 A. Confounding bias
 B. Observer bias
 C. Publication bias
 D. Recall bias
 E. Sampling bias

Answer: B. Observer bias. Blinding in a randomized controlled trial is a method used to minimize potential observer bias.

107. A hospital wants to study the hand hygiene practices of its staff. To gather data, they install cameras to record handwashing in certain areas of the hospital. Once the staff becomes aware of the cameras, a significant increase in handwashing is observed. Which of the following is the most likely issue affecting the study's results?

    A. Confounding bias

    B. Hawthorne effect

    C. Lead-time bias

    D. Observer bias

    E. Selection bias

    Answer: B. Hawthorne effect. In this study, staff who were aware of being monitored by a camera showed an increase in handwashing. This is an example of the Hawthorne effect (observer effect), where individuals modify their behaviour simply because they know they are being observed. This phenomenon can influence the outcomes and potentially undermine the validity of the study.

108. A novel screening test for prostate cancer has been developed, allowing for earlier diagnosis compared to the current standard. In a study, men diagnosed with prostate cancer using the new screening test show a 4-month longer survival than those diagnosed using the traditional methods. However, the study also finds no significant difference in the overall mortality rate between the two groups over a 12-month period. What is the most likely explanation for this finding?

    A. Confounding

    B. Lead-time bias

    C. Length-time bias

    D. Measurement bias

    E. Selection bias

    Answer: B. Lead-time bias. A screening test can identify a disease earlier than a clinical diagnosis, which may misleadingly suggest an increase in survival time without actually improving the prognosis. It's crucial to consider lead-time bias when assessing any screening test. Lead-time bias refers to the false impression of prolonged survival in patients who undergo screening, despite their prognosis remaining unchanged. Patients tested with more sensitive methods might seem to live longer simply because their disease was identified sooner than it would have been with a clinical diagnosis. However, the total time from the onset of the disease to death does not change, whether or not screening occurs.

To accurately evaluate the effectiveness of a screening program, it is important to monitor patients for periods that exceed the perceived increase in survival time, and then to compare mortality rates between those who underwent additional screening and those who did not.

In this particular case, patients evaluated with the new test seemed to have a 4-month longer survival compared to those diagnosed using standard methods. However, there was no difference in the 12-month mortality rates between the two groups, indicating that the screening program does not provide any real benefit.

109. A long-term study investigates the effect of regular aspirin use on the incidence of colorectal cancer. Participants are divided into three groups: those who have taken aspirin daily for less than 3 years, those who have taken aspirin daily for more than 3 years, and those who have never taken aspirin. The results show that individuals who used aspirin for less than 3 years had a relative risk of 1.05 ($p = 0.50$) compared to the non-users, while individuals who used aspirin for more than 3 years had a relative risk of 0.70 ($p < 0.01$). The results of the study were adjusted to account for baseline differences related to healthy behaviors and overall health. What most likely explains the reduced risk of cancer with longer aspirin use?

   A.   Accumulation effect

   B.   Confounding bias

   C.   Lead-time bias

   D.   Recall bias

   E.   Selection bias

Answer: A. Accumulation effect. In this study, the relative risk of colorectal cancer is significantly reduced only in individuals who use aspirin regularly for more than 3 years [RR = 0.70 ($p < 0.01$)]. No association is observed in those using aspirin for less than 3 years [RR = 1.05 ($p = 0.50$)]. This indicates that a longer duration of aspirin exposure (a minimum cumulative exposure) is necessary to observe a significant preventive effect on colorectal cancer development. Accumulation effect is most likely explanation of reduced risk of colorectal cancer with longer aspirin use.

110. Researchers are studying the association between alcohol consumption and lung cancer. They conduct a case-control study by first interviewing a group of patients with biopsy-proven lung cancer and then interviewing a control group of patients without cancer who are admitted for elective surgeries at the same hospital. Both groups are matched on age, gender, and smoking history. This matching technique best helps address which of the following potential problems with this study?

A. Ascertainment bias

B. Confounding

C. Observer bias

D. Recall bias

E. Selection bias

Answer: B. Confounding. Confounding occurs when the relationship between an exposure and a disease is distorted by the influence of a third variable, which is associated with both the exposure and the disease. Techniques like matching, stratification, and randomization help reduce confounding. In this study, cases and controls were matched based on age, gender, and smoking history, ensuring that both groups had similar distributions of potential confounding variables. Matching is a method commonly employed during the design phase of case-control studies to minimize the effects of confounding.

111. Researchers conduct a study to investigate the association between a high-fat diet and the risk of developing colon cancer. The initial analysis finds a relative risk (RR) of 2.5 and a p-value of 0.02, suggesting an increased risk. The researchers then stratify the subjects by exercise habits (active vs. sedentary) and reanalyse the data:

Group	RR	P-value
Active	1.00	0.99
Sedentary	1.05	0.88

The difference between the overall results and the stratified results is best explained by which of the following?
A. Confounding

B. Effect modification

C. Measurement bias

D. Meta-analysis

E. Observer bias

F. Recall bias

Answer: A. Confounding. Confounding occurs when the relationship between an exposure and a disease is distorted by the influence of a third variable, which is associated with both the exposure and the disease. When study subjects are stratified based on this confounding variable, the observed association between the exposure and the disease often disappears.

In this study, the initial crude analysis suggested that a high-fat diet was associated with an increased risk of colon cancer, with a relative risk (RR) of 2.5 and a p-value of 0.02. However, lifestyle factors are linked to both high-fat diet and colon cancer. As a result, lifestyle is a likely confounder that could explain the observed association. After stratifying by activity level, both sedentary and active groups show an RR close to 1, with p-values greater than 0.05, indicating no significant association. The RR of 2.5 found in the crude analysis disappears, suggesting that the original association between high-fat diet and colon cancer was confounded by lifestyle factors.

If this were effect modification, there would be significant differences in the results between strata, indicating a true interaction between variables.

112. A clinical trial is conducted to assess the effect of a new hypertension medication on stroke risk. In men, the medication is associated with a significantly lower risk of stroke (relative risk [RR] = 0.60, p-value = 0.02). However, in women, no significant reduction in stroke risk is observed (RR = 1.05, p-value = 0.75). The researchers note that gender appears to influence the effect of the medication on stroke risk. Which of the following best explains this finding?

    A. Allocation bias

    B. Confounding

    C. Detection bias

    D. Effect modification

    E. Measurement bias

Answer D. Effect modification. Effect modification occurs when the relationship between an exposure and an outcome is altered by another variable. It can be identified through stratified analysis, where the measures of association differ across strata. Unlike confounding, where the measures of association remain similar across strata, effect modification results in a significant difference between them. In this scenario, the outcomes differ between gender strata, indicating the presence of effect modification.

Questions related to intention-to-treat (ITT) analysis

113. A pharmaceutical company is conducting a randomized, double-blind clinical trial to evaluate the effectiveness of enerzair breezhaler, containing indacaterol, glycopyrronium bromide and mometasone for managing uncontrolled asthma. Two hundred patients with poorly controlled asthmatics were randomly assigned to receive either the enerzair breezhaler (n = 100) or standard asthma therapy (n = 100). All participants were instructed to monitor asthma control level using asthma control questionnaire. Changes in treatment plan made according to the trial protocol. After 6 months, 12 participants in the enerzair breezhaler group and 8 in the standard therapy group did not follow the dosing instructions properly. The researchers decide to perform an intention-to-treat analysis. How should the data for patients who did not adhere to the dosing protocol be handled in the ITT analysis?

    A. Analyse all patients as per the group to which they were originally assigned

    B. Analyse patients according to the treatment they actually received

    C. Conduct separate analysis of the 20 non-adherent patients and 180 adherent patients

    D. Exclude non-adherent patients from the analysis

    E. Exclude only patients from the new insulin group

Answer: A. Analyse all patients as per the group to which they were originally assigned. An intention-to-treat (ITT) analysis evaluates treatment groups in a randomized trial by considering all participants in the groups to which they were originally assigned, regardless of their adherence to the study protocol or any events during the trial. This approach assumes that any poor response to treatment, side effects, or noncompliance should still be linked to the assigned treatment, as nonadherence could reflect the practical impact of the intervention. ITT also minimizes the effects of issues like dropout, loss to follow-up, or participants switching to a different treatment, which could compromise the randomization and introduce bias into the study's results.

While ITT analysis often results in a more conservative estimate of the treatment's effectiveness, particularly when there is a significant amount of attrition or crossover, it can make it harder to detect a statistically significant difference between treatments. However, it provides a more accurate reflection of the treatment's expected outcome in real-world clinical practice.

According to ITT principles, in this study, the investigator should analyse all patients as per the their originally assigned groups for analysis.

CHAPTER 1

1. Pediatric pulmonologist monitors the severe asthmatic attack among children who are taking cromolyn sodium, and the finding are plotted as below. What is the average number of severe asthmatic attack per child in one year?

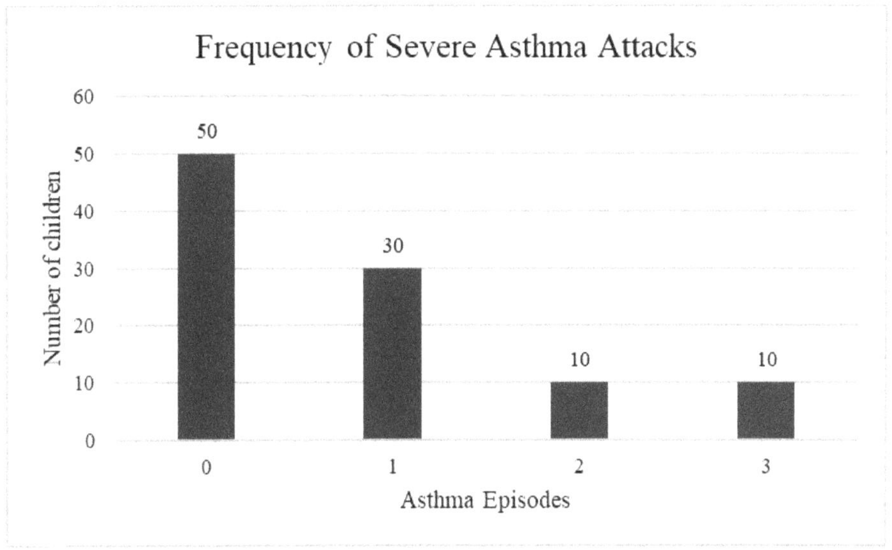

A. Between 0 and 1

B. 1

C. Between 1 and 2

D. 2

E. Between 2 and 3

2. A primary care physician recorded the number of antenatal visits per pregnant mother at his maternal and child health clinic, and the findings are plotted below. What is the average number of antenatal care visits per pregnant mother?

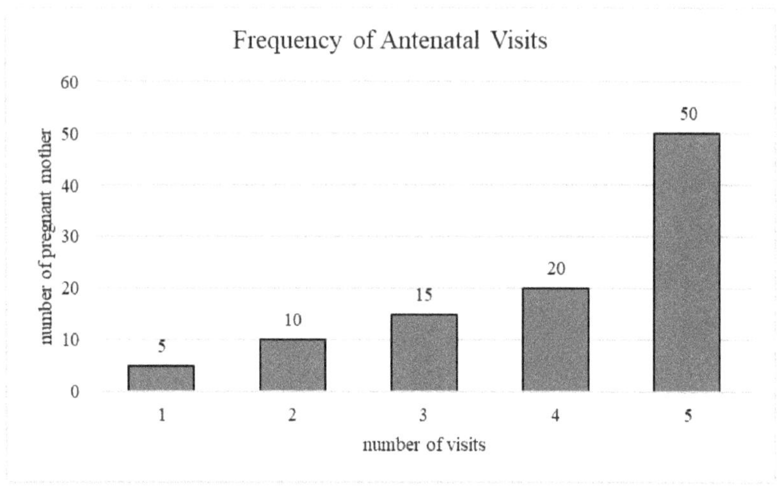

A. Between 2 and 3

B. 3

C. Between 3 and 4

D. 4

E. Between 4 and 5

F. 5

3. A 58-year-old woman with a history of chronic kidney disease is admitted for fluid overload and hypertension. A central venous catheter is placed to monitor her central venous pressure (CVP). Consecutive CVP readings are recorded as follows: 8, 12, 10, 22, 8, and 12 mm Hg. Which of the following represents the median of these CVP readings?

A. 8 mm Hg

B. 10 mm Hg

C. 11 mm Hg

D. 12 mm Hg

E. 22 mm Hg

4. Blood urea nitrogen (BUN) is an important marker used to assess kidney function, with normal levels typically ranging between 7 and 20 mg/dL, measured in whole numbers. A patient in the emergency department had 5 consecutive BUN measurements taken over a 2-hour period. The findings are as follows: 15, 16, 12, 21, 21. Which of the following represents the median BUN level?

    A. 12
    B. 15
    C. 16
    D. 17
    E. 21

5. A patient's heart rate (HR) is being continuously monitored in the intensive care unit. The normal resting heart rate range is between 60-100 beats per minute (bpm), and recorded values are whole numbers. Over a span of 30 minutes, 25 HR readings are recorded. Among these readings, the highest value is 95 bpm and the lowest value is 70 bpm. If the next recorded HR is 120 bpm, which of the following is most likely to remain unchanged?

    A. Median
    B. Mode
    C. Range
    D. Standard deviation
    E. Standard error

6. The hospital director is preparing statistics on the length of stay of admitted patients over the past year. After he made the preparation, one more patient was discharged and his length of stay is 300 days. If he includes this patient's data, which of the following will be unaffected?

    A. Mean
    B. Mode
    C. Range
    D. Standard deviation
    E. Variance

7. An intern collected laboratory data from patients admitted to the ICU and plans to conduct a descriptive analysis of the variables. Blood glucose levels in patients with severe acute pancreatitis were found to have a right-skewed distribution. Which of the following statements is most likely true regarding the data for the severe acute pancreatitis group?

   A. The mean is equal to mode

   B. The mean is greater than median

   C. The mean is not affected

   D. The median is greater than mean

   E. The mode is greater than mean

8. A researcher studies a random sample of 150 women aged 30-40 and finds their average resting heart rate to be 72 beats per minute (bpm), with a standard deviation of 8 bpm. According to national data, resting heart rates for this age group follow a normal (Gaussian) distribution. Based on this information, approximately 68% of women in the sample will have which of the following resting heart rates?

   A. 56-88 bpm

   B. <64 bpm or >80 bpm

   C. 64-80 bpm

   D. <72 bpm

   E. >88 bpm

9. A researcher measures the body mass index (BMI) of 200 randomly selected men aged 40-50, finding the mean BMI to be 26 kg/m², with a standard deviation of 5 kg/m². According to national data, the BMI distribution for men in this age group is approximately normal (Gaussian). Based on this information, approximately 95% of the men in the sample will have which of the following BMI values?

   A. 16-36 kg/m²

   B. <21 kg/m² or >31 kg/m²

   C. 21-31 kg/m²

   D. <26 kg/m²

   E. >36 kg/m²

10. A comprehensive study of fasting blood glucose levels in a group of men aged 25-55 shows a normal distribution with a mean of 90 mg/dL and a standard deviation of 10 mg/dL. According to the study, 99.7% of fasting glucose levels in this population will fall within which of the following ranges?

   A. 60 to 120 mg/dL

   B. 70 to 110 mg/dL

   C. 75 to 105 mg/dL

   D. 80 to 100 mg/dL

   E. 85 to 95 mg/dL

11. A large study analyzing systolic blood pressure in a sample of women aged 35-60 shows a normal distribution with a mean of 120 mmHg and a standard deviation of 10 mmHg. Based on the study findings, 95% of systolic blood pressure values for these women will be within which of the following limits?

   A. 95 to 145 mmHg

   B. 90 to 150 mmHg

   C. 110 to 130 mmHg

   D. 105 to 135 mmHg

   E. 100 to 140 mmHg

12. In a reference sample of several hundred healthy individuals, the laboratory reference range for a new biomarker of kidney function is 0.6-1.0 mg/dL at the standard 95% confidence interval. This biomarker is known for its high sensitivity and specificity for renal tissue. The nephrology team aims to establish a 99.7% reference range to assess patients who come to the clinic with kidney-related symptoms and a high pretest probability of renal impairment. An elevated marker level is defined as exceeding the 99.7th percentile of the reference sample. Assuming a normal (Gaussian) distribution with a mean of 0.8 mg/dL, which of the following best approximates the new cutoff value?

   A. 0.5 mg/dL

   B. 0.6 mg/dL

   C. 0.9 mg/dL

   D. 1.1 mg/dL

   E. 1.2 mg/dL

13. The laboratory reference range for a novel marker indicative of thyroid function is 1.2-1.8 ng/dL at the standard 95% level of confidence. This marker shows very high sensitivity and specificity for thyroid tissue. The endocrinology team would like to adopt a 99.7% reference range to evaluate patients presenting with thyroid dysfunction symptoms and a high pretest probability of thyroid disease. An elevated value of the marker is defined as exceeding the 99.7th percentile of the reference sample. Assuming a normal (Gaussian) distribution with a mean of 1.5 ng/dL, which of the following most closely approximates the corresponding reference range?

    A. 1.05 to 1.95 ng/dL

    B. 1.2 to 1.8 ng/dL

    C. 1.35 to 1.65 ng/dL

    D. 1.4 to 1.6 ng/dL

    E. 1.45 to 1.55 ng/dL

14. Body mass index (BMI) measurements were collected from a sample of individuals with no known medical conditions. The mean BMI values and associated standard deviations (SDs) for different age groups in men and women are displayed below:

Men		Women	
Age	Mean BMI (kg/m^2) ± SD	Age	Mean BMI (kg/m^2) ± SD
35-44	26 ± 4	35-44	25 ± 3
45-54	28 ± 5	45-54	27 ± 4
55-64	30 ± 6	55-64	29 ± 5

    If obesity is defined as a BMI greater than 30 kg/m^2, what percentage of men aged 55-64 in this sample would likely be classified as obese, assuming a normal (Gaussian) distribution?

    A. 15%

    B. 30%

    C. 50%

    D. 70%

    E. 85%

15. A sample of individuals with no known medical conditions was analyzed for fasting blood glucose levels. The mean glucose levels and corresponding standard deviations (SDs) for men and women by age group are summarized below:

Men		Women	
Age	Mean Glucose (mg/dL) ± SD	Age	Mean Glucose (mg/dL) ± SD
35-44	90 ± 10	35-44	88 ± 9
45-54	100 ± 12	45-54	95 ± 11
55-64	110 ± 14	55-64	105 ± 13

If diabetes is defined as fasting blood glucose levels exceeding 112 mg/dL, what percentage of men aged 45-54 in this sample would likely be classified as not having diabetes, assuming a normal (Gaussian) distribution?

A. 16%

B. 50%

C. 68%

D. 84%

E. 95%

16. A research study evaluated the age at which adolescents begin smoking cigarettes. Participants were categorized into two groups: regular smokers and occasional smokers.

Smoker Type	Sample Size (n)	Mean Age (years)	Standard Deviation (years)
Regular	40	14.8	1.2
Occasional	35	17.0	1.5

Assuming that the age at which smoking begins is normally distributed, what is the probability that a randomly selected regular smoker will start smoking at age 16 or younger?

A. 0.025

B. 0.050

C. 0.840

D. 0.950

E. 0.975

17. A survey was conducted to assess the age at which individuals begin drinking alcohol. Respondents were divided into two categories: frequent drinkers and occasional drinkers.

Drinker Type	Sample Size (n)	Mean Age (years)	Standard Deviation (years)
Frequent	50	18.4	1.6
Occasional	45	20.0	1.2

Assuming that the age at which individuals start drinking is normally distributed, what is the probability that a randomly chosen frequent drinker will have their first drink at age 20 or older?

A. 0.025

B. 0.050

C. 0.160

D. 0.320

E. 0.950

18. An intern in the nephrology unit is assigned to analyze kidney function tests for all patients hospitalized due to chronic kidney disease (CKD) in the last six months. The intern finds that there were 200 patients, and the estimated glomerular filtration rate (eGFR) levels were normally distributed with a mean of 60 mL/min and a standard deviation of 15 mL/min. Based on this information, how many patients in this study would likely have an eGFR <45 mL/min?

A. 5

B. 10

C. 16

D. 32

E. 50

19. A medical officer in the gastroenterology department is reviewing liver enzyme levels of all patients admitted with liver-related complications over the past six months. The preliminary analysis shows that there were 100 patients, with serum alanine aminotransferase (ALT) levels normally distributed, a mean of 45 U/L, and a standard deviation of 5 U/L. How many patients in this study would be expected to have ALT levels ≥ 55 U/L?

    A.   <1

    B.   5

    C.   10

    D.   16

    E.   34

20. An epidemiologist is researching the serum ferritin levels in women of reproductive age living in a community with a high prevalence of iron deficiency anemia. She takes a large random sample of women aged 18-40 and measures their serum ferritin levels. The data show a normal distribution, with the mean and standard deviation (SD) reported. To assess sampling variation, she computes a 95% confidence interval to estimate the mean ferritin level in the broader population. The epidemiologist concludes that the true population mean is likely between 12 and 18 ng/mL. Which of the following calculations was most likely utilized to compute this interval estimate for the population mean?

    A.   Mean $\pm (SD/\sqrt{n})$

    B.   Mean $\pm 1.96 \times (SD/\sqrt{n})$

    C.   Mean $\pm 1.96 \times SD$

    D.   Mean $\pm 2.58 \times (SD/\sqrt{n})$

    E.   Mean $\pm 2.58 \times SD$

CHAPTER 2

21. A biotech firm creates a new genetic screening test for a hereditary heart condition. When compared to genetic sequencing, which is the most accurate diagnostic method, the new test correctly identifies 90% of individuals who do not have the condition as negative. If this test is applied to a group of 5 individuals who are known to be free of the condition, what is the probability that all 5 results will be negative?

   A. 0.10×5

   B. 0.10^5

   C. 0.90×5

   D. 0.90^5

   E. $1 - 0.10^5$

   F. $1 - 0.90^5$

22. A healthcare provider develops a new rapid test for detecting a bacterial infection. Compared to bacterial culture, the new test correctly identifies 85% of patients without the infection as negative. If the test is administered to 7 individuals who are confirmed not to have the infection, what is the probability that all 7 tests will yield a positive result?

   A. 0.15×7

   B. 0.85×7

   C. 0.15^7

   D. 0.85^7

   E. $1 - 0.15^7$

   F. $1 - 0.85^7$

23. A public health team is assessing the prevalence of high cholesterol in an urban neighborhood. The estimated prevalence rates (cases per 100 individuals) for different age and gender groups are provided below:

Age Group	Women	Men
40-49	18.0	20.0
50-59	25.0	30.0
60-69	32.0	35.0
70+	40.0	45.0
Total	29.0	32.5

In one afternoon, a doctor sees a 55-year-old woman, a 67-year-old man, and a 73-year-old woman from this neighborhood. Assuming the probability of high cholesterol for each individual is independent, what is the probability that none of them has high cholesterol?

A. 0.035

B. 0.038

C. 0.102

D. 0.293

E. 0.333

24. A group of evolutionary biologists is investigating the frequency of coat color alleles in a population of wild rabbits. They have recorded the following genotypic distribution among 50 rabbits: 20 CC (brown coat), 20 Cc (brown coat), and 10 cc (white coat). Coat color does not affect the rabbits' survival or reproductive success. The rabbits breed freely in a large forested area, with no new individuals entering or leaving the population. Based on these observations, is the allele and genotype distribution in this rabbit population in Hardy-Weinberg equilibrium?

A. No, because coat color is not under selective pressure.

B. No, because the genotype distribution does not reflect expected proportions.

C. No, because the sample size is relatively small.

D. Yes, because random mating and a stable environment support equilibrium.

25. A group of biologists is studying a population of 20 birds in a forest to track the distribution of a feather color gene. The genotype distribution in the population is 6 BB (dark feathers), 8 Bb (intermediate feathers), and 6 bb (light feathers). The forest was recently divided by a natural disaster, isolating the population from other bird groups. Birds within the population mate randomly. Based on the information provided, is this population in Hardy-Weinberg equilibrium for the feather color gene?

    A.   No, because the population size is too small

    B.   No, because there is no migration or gene flow into the population

    C.   Yes, because the birds mate randomly

    D.   Yes, because the feather color does not affect survival

26. In a study of a rabbit population living on an island, researchers observed the following genotype distribution for ear size: 12 EE (large ears), 5 Ee (medium ears), and 3 ee (small ears). The population size has been declining due to a shortage of food, and the researchers noticed that rabbits with larger ears are better at finding food and surviving. The island's population is isolated from outside rabbit populations, and the rabbits mate randomly. Based on this information, are the allele and genotype frequencies in this population in Hardy-Weinberg equilibrium?

    A.   No, because the population is not large and randomly mating

    B.   No, because there is selection favoring one genotype over others

    C.   Yes, because the population is isolated with no migration

    D.   Yes, because the rabbits mate randomly

27. A 34-year-old woman and her husband are considering having their first child. She is a known carrier of Tay-Sachs disease, a rare autosomal recessive disorder that affects approximately 1 in 250,000 individuals. Her husband has no known family history of the disease, but his carrier status is not determined. What is the probability that their child will be affected by Tay-Sachs disease?

    A.   1/4

    B.   1/500

    C.   1/1,000

    D.   1/2,000

    E.   1/250,000

28. A 30-year-old man and his wife are planning to have a second child. The couple's first child was diagnosed with phenylketonuria (PKU), an autosomal recessive disorder occurring in approximately 1 in 10,000 individuals. Genetic testing confirms that both parents are carriers of the disorder. They are concerned about the risk of having another child with PKU. What is the probability that their next child will be affected by PKU?

A. 1/4

B. 1/10

C. 1/40

D. 1/100

E. 1/10,000

29. A team of zoologists is analysing a specific gene in a population of wild horses. This gene has two allelic forms, E and F. Horses with EE and EF genotypes show the dominant characteristic, while horses with the FF genotype show the recessive phenotype. The population size is 400, and the following genotype distribution has been documented:

Genotype	Number of Frogs
EE	150
EF	180
FF	70

Which of the following represents the frequency of the F allele in this horse population?

A. 70/400

B. 180/400

C. 250/400

D. 250/800

E. 320/800

F. 480/800

30. In a study of a specific gene in a population of birds, researchers are focusing on two alleles, G and H. Birds with GG and GH genotypes display the dominant trait, while those with the HH genotype display the recessive trait. In a population of 600 birds, the genotype distribution is as follows:

Genotype	Number of Frogs
GG	240
GH	270
HH	90

What is the frequency of the G allele in this population?

A. 90/600

B. 360/600

C. 510/600

D. 450/1200

E. 540/1200

F. 750/1200

CHAPTER 3

31. Researchers are analyzing the incidence and prevalence of hospital-acquired pressure ulcers in the surgical ward of a regional hospital. The chart below illustrates the daily count of patients diagnosed with pressure ulcers throughout the month of March. Using the information provided, what is the number of incident cases for the month of March?

A. 3

B. 4

C. 5

D. 7

E. 11

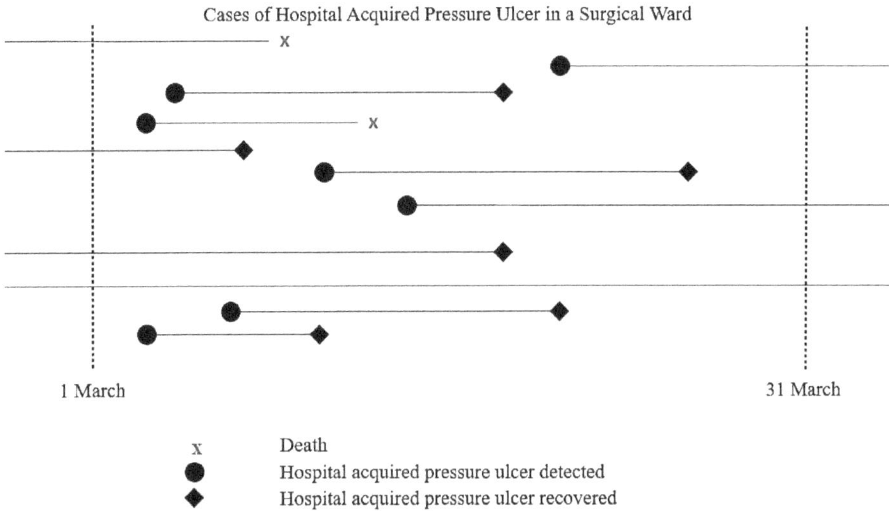

32. In 2020, a country with a population of 10,000,000 reported 50,000 cases of a newly discovered chronic illness at the start of the year. By year's end, 20,000 more cases were identified, and 2,000 individuals had died from this illness. Additionally, 78,000 deaths from other causes were recorded. What is the cumulative incidence of this illness for the year 2020?

A. 2,000 / 78,000

B. 20,000 / 9,920,000

C. 20,000 / 9,950,000

D. 20,000 / 10,000,000

E. 70,000 / 9,920,000

F. F70,000 / 10,000,000

33. A coastal city has a population of 2,200,000 people as of 2022. At the start of the year, the city had 20,000 cases of a chronic respiratory disease due to long-term exposure to air pollution. By the end of the year, 3,000 new cases of the disease were reported, and 500 individuals died from the condition. Additionally, there were 10,000 deaths from all other causes. What is the cumulative incidence of the chronic respiratory disease in 2022?

A. 500 / 2,200,000

B. 3,500 / 2,180,000

C. 3,500 / 2,200,000

D. 3,000 / 2,180,000

E. 3,000 / 2,200,000

F. 23,000 / 2,185,000

34. A corporate office hosted a luncheon where sandwiches, salad, and pasta were served. Out of the 150 employees who attended, 40 reported symptoms of abdominal cramps and diarrhoea the following day. Employees were surveyed about what they ate, and the following table was obtained:

Food item or combination of items	Number of attendees who ate food item or combination of items	Number of attendees who developed symptoms
Sandwiches only	30	6
Salad only	20	4
Pasta only	15	1
Sandwiches and salad	35	10
Sandwiches and pasta	10	3
Salad and pasta	15	6
Sandwiches, salad, and pasta	25	10

Which of the following best describes the attack rate among all attendees who had sandwiches?

    A. 7%

    B. 15%

    C. 20%

    D. 25%

    E. 29%

    F. 30%

    G. 40%

    H. 50%

35. A high school held an end-of-year picnic where pizza, fruit salad, and ice cream were served. The next day, 50 of the 200 students who attended reported stomach pain and nausea. The students were asked what they had eaten, and the following table was compiled:

Food item or combination of items	Number of attendees who ate food item or combination of items	Number of attendees who developed symptoms
Pizza only	40	5
Fruit salad only	30	2
Ice cream only	25	1
Pizza and fruit salad	40	12
Pizza and ice cream	30	7
Fruit salad and ice cream	20	6
Pizza, fruit salad, and ice cream	15	4

Which of the following best describes the attack rate among all attendees who had ice cream?

A. 12%

B. 15%

C. 18%

D. 20%

E. 28%

F. 32%

G. 35%

H. 40%

36. A university hospital reviews its outcomes for sepsis cases admitted to its intensive care unit (ICU). The table below presents the sepsis-related mortality for the past year:

Infection Type	Number of Fatal Cases	% of All Fatal Cases	Number of Nonfatal Cases	% of All Nonfatal Cases
E. coli	15	20	60	30
P. aeruginosa	25	33	40	20
S. aureus*, methicillin-resistant	30	40	50	25
S. aureus*, methicillin-sensitive	5	7	30	15
Other	0	0	20	10
Total	75	100	200	100

What is the case-fatality rate for *P. aeruginosa* sepsis in this hospital?

A. 25/40

B. 25/65

C. 25/75

D. 25/200

E. 40/200

37. A major urban hospital is conducting an audit of its nosocomial (hospital-acquired) infections over the past year. The mortality data for various nosocomial bloodstream infections are summarized below:

Infection Type	Number of fatal cases	% of all fatal Cases	Number of nonfatal Cases	% of All nonfatal Cases
Candida species	30	38	80	35
E. coli	10	12	40	18
Enterococcus species	5	6	30	13
MRSA	20	25	50	22
Other	15	19	30	13
Total	80	100	230	100

What is the case-fatality rate for *Candida* infections in this hospital?

A. 30/80

B. 30/110

C. 30/230

D. 38/100

E. 80/230

38. A certain viral infection, which affects primarily children, has shown consistent prevalence in a population over the last 10 years. Recently, a mass vaccination program was introduced, significantly reducing the transmission of the virus. Assuming other conditions remain constant, what is the most likely impact on the prevalence of the infection in the population?

A. It is not possible to determine the effect on prevalence from the information given

B. The prevalence would decrease

C. The prevalence would increase

D. The prevalence would remain the same

39. In a population with a consistent prevalence of diabetes, a new fast-food chain opens, offering unhealthy food at very low prices. Over the next few years, a large proportion of the population starts consuming more unhealthy food, while the healthcare system and treatment options remain unchanged. What is the most likely effect of this change on the prevalence of diabetes in the population?

A. It is not possible to determine the effect on prevalence from the information given

B. The prevalence would decrease

C. The prevalence would increase

D. The prevalence would remain the same

40. A study reported the number of Brazilian women living with breast cancer, illustrated in the following figure. Assuming the Brazilian population is stable, which of the following is the most likely explanation for the changes in disease prevalence depicted in the graph?

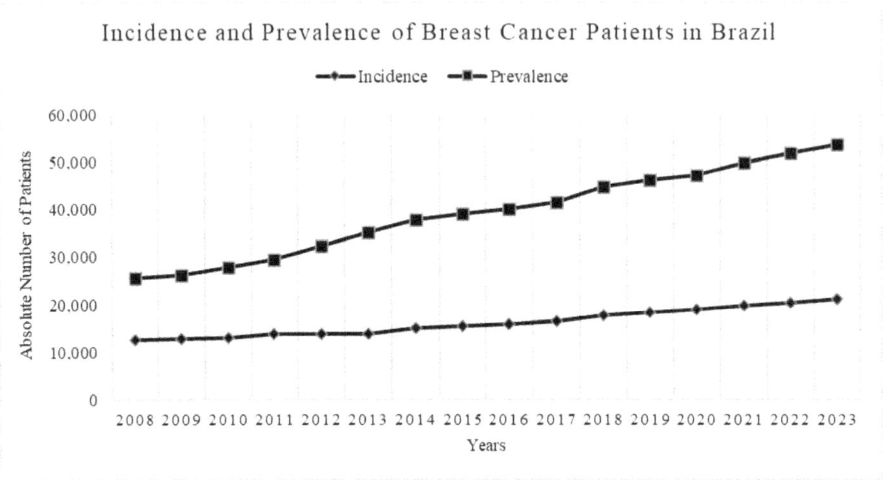

A. Reduced hospitalization rates

B. Elevated mortality from diabetes

C. Improved quality of care

D. Greater precision in diagnostic testing

E. Higher exposure to risk factors

F. Rise in the number of new diabetes cases

G. Survival bias due to selective factors

41. A population-based study of breast cancer prevalence in Australia reported the following graph of breast cancer incidence and mortality from 1972 to 2007. Based on the figure, what is the prediction of breast cancer situation in 2017.

A. The number of incident cases will decrease in 2017

B. The number of deaths will increase in 2017

C. The number of prevalent cases will decrease in 2017

D. The number of prevalent cases will increase in 2017

E. The number of prevalent cases will remain unchanged in 2017

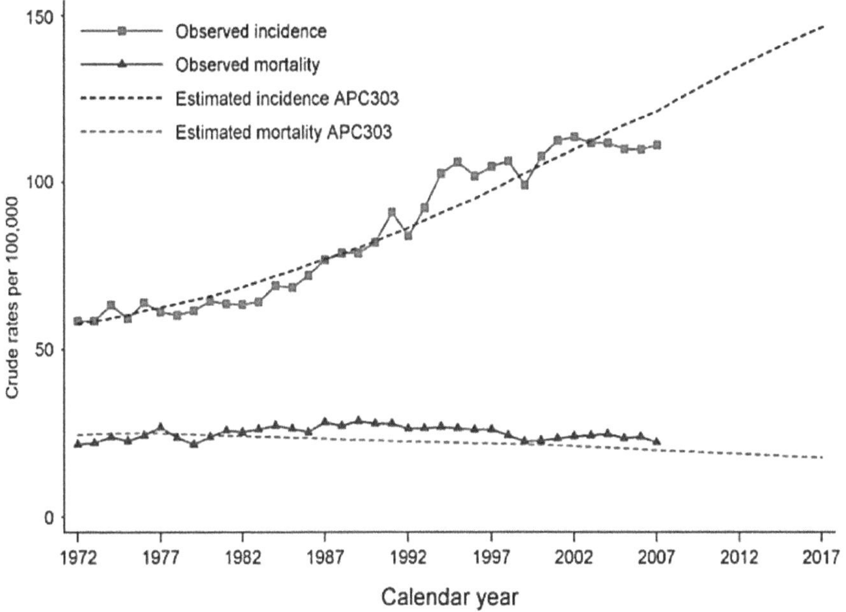

Source: Yu, X.Q., De Angelis, R., Luo, Q. et al. A population-based study of breast cancer prevalence in Australia: predicting the future health care needs of women living with breast cancer. BMC Cancer 14, 936 (2014).

42. A 65-year-old man is diagnosed with end-stage kidney disease (ESKD). A new dialysis technology is introduced that significantly increases the life expectancy of ESKD patients but does not cure the underlying condition. If this technology is widely adopted, how would it affect the number of incident and prevalent cases of ESKD?

A. The number of incident cases will decrease

B. The number of incident cases will increase

C. The number of prevalent cases will decrease

D. The number of prevalent cases will increase

E. The number of prevalent cases will remain unchanged

43. A pharmaceutical company develops a new medication for patients with severe heart failure that slows the progression of the disease and prolongs life but does not cure it. If this medication becomes widely used, what would be the expected effect on the incidence and prevalence of heart failure in the population?

A. The number of incident cases will decrease, the number of prevalent cases will decrease

B. The number of incident cases will decrease, the number of prevalent cases will increase

C. The number of incident cases will increase, the number of prevalent cases will remain unchanged

D. The number of incident cases will not change, the number of prevalent cases will increase

E. The number of incident cases will not change, the number of prevalent cases will remain unchanged

44. The population pyramid of Afghanistan is shown below.

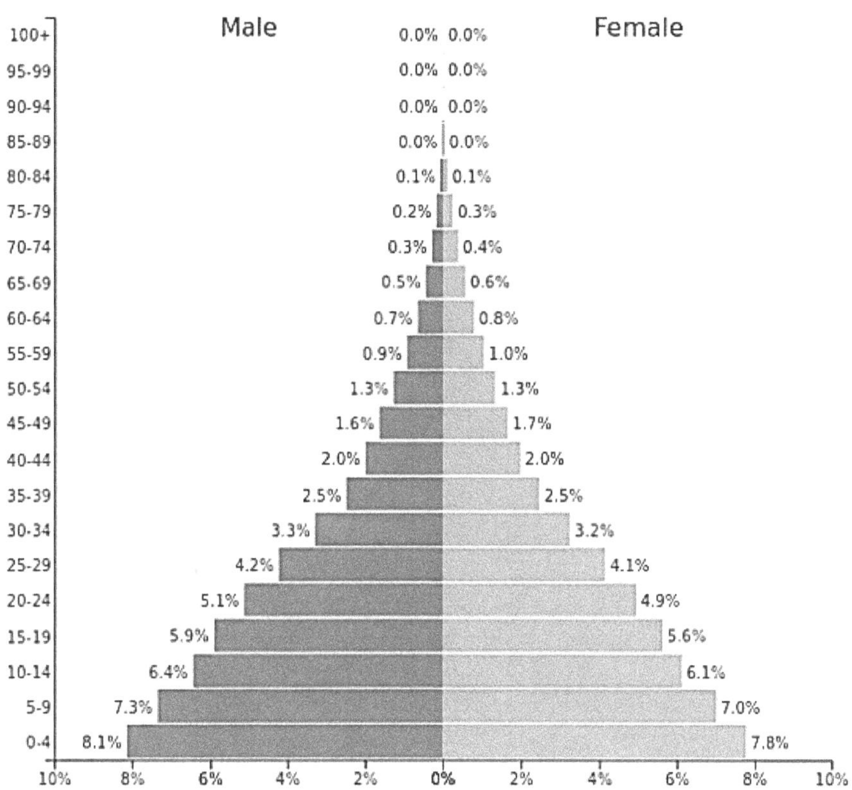

Based on the diagram, which of the following best characterized this population?

A. High mortality

B. Long life expectance

C. Low birth rate

D. Shrinking population

E. Sable population

45. Which of the following statements best describe the population of Myanmar?

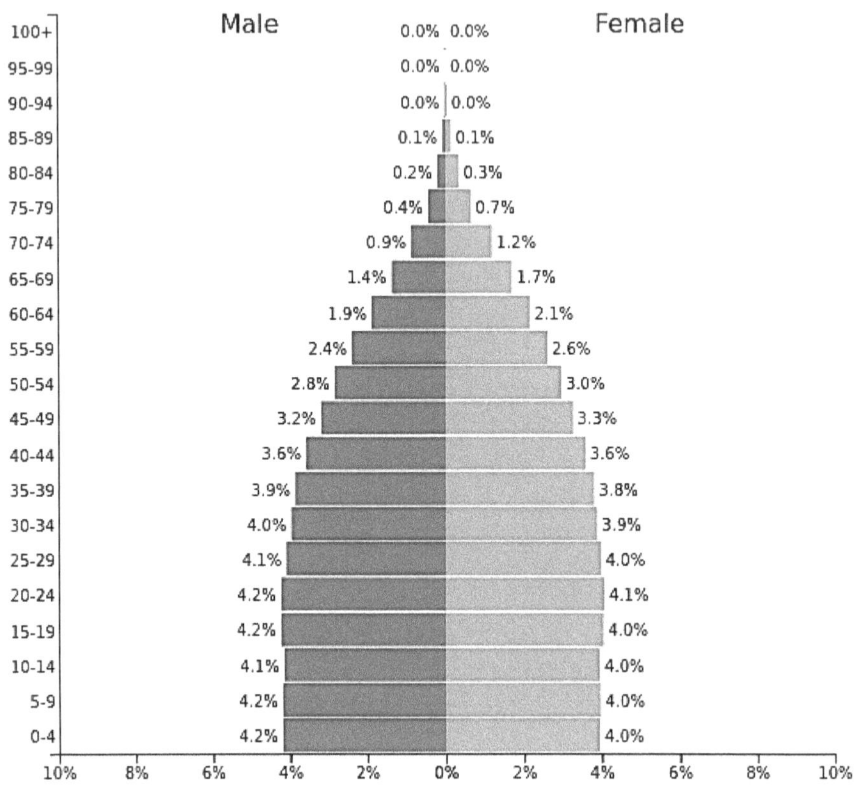

A. High birth rate indicates the population is growing

B. Myanmar has a young population because of its high birth rate

C. Population consists of older group of people compared to young.

D. The population is shrinking due to the migration of old people

E. The similar number of people in each age cohort indicates the population is stable

CHAPTER 4

46. A dermatologist is interested in documenting the clinical characteristics of a rare skin condition. The researcher gathers information from 7 patients diagnosed with the condition, focusing on their skin biopsy results, treatment regimens, and disease progression over time. No interventions or control groups are involved. What is the most appropriate description of this study design?

A. Case series

B. Case-control study

C. Clinical trial

D. Cohort

E. Cross-sectional

47. A cardiology research team studies 12 patients who experienced severe side effects after receiving a new medication for heart disease. The study describes their medical history, the side effects they encountered, and the steps taken to manage these adverse reactions. No comparisons are made with other patients, and no treatments are tested. Which of the following best describes this study design?

A. Case series

B. Clinical trial

C. Cohort

D. Cross over study

E. Cross-sectional

48. Researchers are studying the relationship between obesity and sleep disorders in a population. They randomly select participants from various regions and record their body mass index (BMI) and current sleep patterns using a standardized questionnaire. All data is assessed at one time, and the researchers aim to explore the association between BMI and the occurrence of sleep disorders. Which of the following best describes this study design?

A. Case-control study

B. Cross-sectional study

    C. Prospective cohort study

    D. Randomized clinical trial

    E. Retrospective cohort study

49. A team of public health scientists is exploring the link between vaping and depressive symptoms in adolescents. They conduct a survey in which students from multiple high schools are asked about their vaping habits and whether they currently experience depressive symptoms such as feeling sadness, low self-esteem, tiredness or changes in appetite. The researchers analyze this data to identify any associations, but the information is only collected at a single point in time. Which of the following best describes the study design?

    A. Case-control study

    B. Cross-sectional study

    C. Ecological Study

    D. Prospective cohort study

    E. Randomized clinical trial

50. A group of researchers is studying the relationship between different types of diet and colon cancer. They recruit 30 patients recently diagnosed with colon cancer and 60 patients without cancer from the same hospital. The researchers ask all participants to complete a detailed dietary history to assess their dietary phenol consumption over the past 10 years. Which of the following best describes this study design?

    A. Case series study

    B. Case-control study

    C. Cross-sectional study

    D. Prospective cohort study

    E. Randomized control trial

51. Researchers aim to investigate the potential link between long-term use of proton pump inhibitors (PPIs) and the development of osteoporosis. They select 100 patients recently diagnosed with osteoporosis and match them with 100 patients without osteoporosis from the same healthcare system. The researchers review medical records to determine each patient's history of PPI use over the past 5 years. Which of the following best describes the study design used by the researchers?
    A. Case-control study
    B. Cross-sectional study
    C. Prospective cohort study
    D. Randomized controlled trial
    E. Retrospective cohort study

52. Investigators are examining the association between frequent use of mobile phones and brain tumors. They identify 25 patients with newly diagnosed brain tumors and 50 individuals without tumors from the same neurology clinic. They interview participants about their mobile phone usage over the last 5 years to assess exposure. Which of the following best describes this study design?
    A. Case series study
    B. Case-control study
    C. Cross-sectional study
    D. Prospective cohort study
    E. Randomized control trial

53. A team of researchers is exploring the possible link between high coffee consumption and bladder cancer. They recruit 50 patients recently diagnosed with bladder cancer and 100 healthy participants without bladder cancer from the same region. The researchers use questionnaires to collect data on the participants' coffee drinking habits over the last 20 years. Which of the following Best describes this study design?
    A. Case-cohort study
    B. Case-control study
    C. Case-series study
    D. Cohort study
    E. Cross-sectional study

54. Investigators are studying whether there is an association between shift work and the development of cardiovascular disease. They select 150 individuals without cardiovascular disease from local hospitals and categorize them into two groups: 75 individuals who have worked night shifts over the past 10 years and 75 who have not. Both groups are followed over time to assess the incidence of cardiovascular disease. Which of the following best describes this study design?

   A. Case-cohort study

   B. Case-control study

   C. Case-series study

   D. Cohort study

   E. Cross-sectional study

55. In 1998, a researcher enrolled 3,000 pregnant women to investigate the effects of prenatal exposure to air pollution on child development. The women were categorized based on their exposure to air pollution during pregnancy. Their children were then monitored for cognitive and physical developmental milestones up to the age of 10. The data was compared between children exposed to high levels of pollution and those exposed to low levels. What is the MOST appropriate study design for this research?

   A. Case-control study

   B. Case-series study

   C. Cohort study

   D. Cross-sectional study

   E. Ecological study

56. A health researcher is analyzing the relationship between physical activity and the risk of developing diabetes. In 2010, the researcher recruited 6,000 participants aged 30-50, divided into those who regularly engage in physical activity and those who lead a sedentary lifestyle. Over a 12-year period, the participants were assessed annually to track the onset of diabetes and other disorders. What is the most appropriate study design for this research?

A. Case-control study

B. Cohort study

C. Cross-sectional study

D. Ecological study

E. Randomized clinical trial

57. In 2021, a group of researchers aimed to investigate the impact of childhood exposure to second-hand smoke on the development of asthma in adulthood. They reviewed the medical records of 1,500 individuals born between 1975 and 1995, categorizing them into two groups based on the exposure to second-hand smoke as children. The researchers then analyzed health outcomes from 1995 to 2021 to determine the incidence of asthma and other respiratory conditions. Which of the following best describes the study design?

A. Case-control study

B. Cross-sectional study

C. Prospective cohort study

D. Randomized clinical trial

E. Retrospective cohort study

58. A study was conducted in 2019 to assess the long-term effects of prenatal exposure to alcohol on children's cognitive development. The researchers examined the medical and educational records of 800 children born between 1990 and 2005. These children were divided into groups based on their mothers' reported alcohol consumption during pregnancy. Cognitive test scores from 2005 to 2019 were analyzed to determine the impact of prenatal alcohol exposure. Which of the following best describes the study design?

   A. Case-control study

   B. Cross-sectional study

   C. Prospective cohort study

   D. Randomized clinical trial

   E. Retrospective cohort study

59. A study is conducted to investigate whether certain agricultural practices are associated with higher rates of chronic kidney disease (CKD). Researchers gathered data on the percentage of agricultural land using synthetic fertilizers in various regions, along with the CKD prevalence rates reported by regional health agencies. The analysis aimed to determine if regions with higher use of synthetic fertilizers had higher rates of CKD. Which of the following best describes the design of this study?

   A. Case-control study

   B. Cohort study

   C. Cross-sectional study

   D. Ecological study

   E. Randomized controlled trial

60. A study is conducted to assess the impact of urbanization on cardiovascular disease rates. Researchers obtained data on the percentage of urban populations from various countries, as well as the national cardiovascular disease mortality rates reported by each country's health ministry. The analysis aimed to determine if countries with a higher percentage of urban residents had higher cardiovascular mortality rates. Which of the following best describes the design of this study?

A. Case-control study

B. Clinical trial

C. Cohort study

D. Cross-sectional study

E. Ecological study

61. A research team is investigating the effectiveness of a new cognitive-behavioral therapy (CBT) program in reducing symptoms of anxiety in college students. One hundred students diagnosed with anxiety disorders are randomly assigned to either receive the new CBT program or standard counseling sessions. Both groups undergo therapy for 12 weeks, and their anxiety levels are measured at the start and end of the treatment using standardized anxiety scales. The outcomes of the two groups are then compared. Which of the following best describes the study design?

A. Case-control study

B. Crossover design

C. Prospective cohort study

D. Randomized controlled trial

E. Retrospective cohort study

62. A pharmaceutical company is testing the effectiveness of baxdrostat, a selective aldosterone synthase inhibitor, to reduce high blood pressure. A total of 300 participants with diagnosed hypertension are randomly assigned to receive either baxdrostat or a placebo. Both groups take their respective pills daily for 6 months, and their blood pressure is measured weekly. At the end of the study, the results from both groups are compared to determine the drug's effectiveness. Which of the following best describes the study design?

    A. Case-control study

    B. Cross-sectional study

    C. Cross-over study

    D. Prospective cohort study

    E. Randomized controlled trial

63. A study aims to investigate the effectiveness of nasal spray influenza vaccine in the prevention seasonal influenza. Two thousand participants are randomly divided into two groups: one group receives the nasal spray influenza vaccine, and the other receives a placebo. Both groups are monitored throughout the flu season, and the number of confirmed flu cases in each group is recorded and compared. Which of the following best describes the study design?

    A. Case-control study

    B. Crossover design

    C. Prospective cohort study

    D. Randomized controlled trial

    E. Retrospective cohort study

64. Researchers want to determine the effect of two different diets (a high-protein diet and a low-protein diet) on weight loss in individuals with obesity. Forty participants are randomly divided into two groups: one group follows the high-protein diet for six weeks, and the other follows the low-protein diet. After a two-week washout period, the participants switch diets for another six weeks. Weight is measured before and after each diet phase. Which of the following best describes this study design?

A. Case-control study

B. Crossover design

C. Prospective cohort study

D. Randomized controlled trial

E. Retrospective cohort study

65. A study is conducted to evaluate the impact of two different inhalers (Relvar Ellipta inhaler or placebo inhaler) on asthma symptom control in patients. Twenty-five patients are randomly assigned to receive the steroid inhaler for four weeks, followed by a placebo inhaler for another four weeks, with a one-week washout period in between. After each treatment phase, patients complete a symptom severity questionnaire. Which of the following best describes this study design?

A. Case-control study

B. Crossover study

C. Cross-sectional study

D. Prospective cohort study

E. Randomized controlled trial

66. Researchers assess the safety and pharmacokinetics of a new antiviral compound, Viralyn, designed to inhibit viral replication. The study involves 24 healthy adults voluneers, each receiving a single oral dose ranging from 10 to 100 mg/kg. The goal is to track drug absorption and elimination while monitoring for adverse effects. Initial results show Viralyn is well tolerated at all doses, with no serious adverse events, though mild nausea is reported in three participants at the highest dose. Which of the following best describes this study?

A. Preclinical study

B. Phase I clinical trial

C. Phase II clinical trial

D. Phase III clinical trial

E. Phase IV clinical trial

67. Researchers are investigating the safety profile of a new anti-cancer agent, Tumorinib, in a trial involving 15 healthy volunteers. The participants receive escalating doses of Tumorinib via intravenous infusion, starting from 0.25 mg/kg up to 20 mg/kg. The primary endpoints are to determine the maximum tolerated dose and document any early signs of toxicity. Volunteers are also monitored for pharmacokinetic parameters, including clearance rates and drug distribution in the bloodstream. So far, Tumorinib has demonstrated no severe side effects. Mild and reversible skin rashes occur in two subjects at higher doses, but no significant toxicities are reported. Which of the following best describes this type of study?

A. Preclinical study

B. Phase I clinical trial

C. Phase II clinical trial

D. Phase III clinical trial

E. Phase IV clinical trial

68. As part of a clinical investigation for imeglimin, a new diabetes medication, researchers evaluate its effectiveness in controlling blood sugar levels. Seventy patients with Type 2 diabetes are randomized into four groups: one receiving a placebo and three others receiving different doses of the drug. After 12 weeks, results show a dose-dependent improvement in glucose control, with the highest dose reducing HbA1c levels the most but causing more hypoglycemia. Researchers conclude that the medium dose offers the best balance between efficacy and safety. Which of the following best describes this study?

A. Preclinical study

B. Phase I clinical trial

C. Phase II clinical trial

D. Phase III clinical trial

E. Phase IV clinical trial

69. Peresolimab, a humanized IgG1 monoclonal antibody, stimulates the PD-1 inhibitory pathway, offering a novel approach for treating autoimmune diseases. Researchers test its role in rheumatoid arthritis patients who haven't responded to conventional treatments. In this trial, 80 patients are randomized to receive either standard medication with placebo or standard medication plus one of two doses of peresolimab. Over six months, patients are assessed for improvements in joint inflammation, pain, and physical function. The higher dose shows better reductions in swelling but more side effects, while the lower dose offers a better balance of benefits and risks. Which of the following best describes this study?

A. Preclinical study

B. Phase I clinical trial

C. Phase II clinical trial

D. Phase III clinical trial

E. Phase IV clinical trial

70. A pharmaceutical company tests baxdrostat, a selective aldosterone synthase inhibitor, against an existing antihypertensive in a large international study. 1,200 patients with hypertension are randomized to receive either baxdrostat or the leading medication. Over one year, patients are monitored for changes in blood pressure and cardiovascular events like heart attacks and strokes. The new drug significantly reduces blood pressure but shows a slight increase in dizziness and fatigue in some patients. Which of the following best describes this study?

    A. Preclinical study

    B. Phase I clinical trial

    C. Phase II clinical trial

    D. Phase III clinical trial

    E. Phase IV clinical trial

71. Researchers are conducting a clinical trial to test the efficacy of a new vaccine for preventing respiratory syncytial virus (RSV) in the elderly. 3,000 older adults from multiple centers are randomized into two groups: one receiving the vaccine and the other a placebo. Over two years, participants are monitored for RSV infections and serious side effects. The vaccine significantly reduces RSV infections compared to the placebo, with only minor side effects like mild injection site reactions. Which of the following best describes this study?

    A. Preclinical study

    B. Phase I clinical trial

    C. Phase II clinical trial

    D. Phase III clinical trial

    E. Phase IV clinical trial

72. A post-marketing surveillance study is conducted to monitor the long-term safety and efficacy of a new oral anticoagulant used for stroke prevention in patients with atrial fibrillation. 10,500 patients with atrial fibrillation are enrolled, and they receive the anticoagulant for 12 months. The study results indicate effective stroke prevention, but an unexpected increase in gastrointestinal bleeding is observed in 72 patients, particularly those with a history of peptic ulcers. Based on these findings, the publication suggests that gastroprotective agents should be co-prescribed for patients

with a high risk of gastrointestinal bleeding. Which of the following best characterizes this type of study?

A. Phase I clinical trial

B. Phase II clinical trial

C. Phase III clinical trial

D. Phase IV clinical trial

E. Preclinical study

73. A long-term safety study is carried out on a recently approved inhaled corticosteroid for managing chronic obstructive pulmonary disease (COPD). 7,200 patients with moderate to severe COPD are enrolled and treated with the drug over two years. While the drug shows sustained improvements in lung function, bone density loss is detected in 112 patients, leading to a rise in fractures. The study concludes that patients with osteoporosis or other bone health risks may require regular bone density monitoring and possible treatment adjustments. Which of the following best characterizes this type of study?

A. Preclinical study

B. Phase I clinical trial

C. Phase II clinical trial

D. Phase III clinical trial

E. Phase IV clinical trial

74. A public health researcher is investigating the risk factors associated with the development of Type 2 diabetes in a population with high obesity rates. She assembles a case-control study involving a cohort of adults diagnosed with Type 2 diabetes and a cohort of age-matched, diabetes-free adults. Her primary goal is to evaluate the relationship between dietary habits, such as high sugar intake, and the incidence of diabetes. Which of the following would be the most appropriate measure of interest for this study?

A. Frequency of sugary food consumption in each cohort

B. Incidence of diabetic complications in the cases

C. Rate of exercise in the control group

D. Rate of insulin use among participants

E. The average fasting blood glucose levels in each cohort

75. A cardiologist conducts a study to compare the effectiveness of two blood pressure medications, Aprocitentan and Losartan, in preventing heart attacks. He enrolls 1,500 patients with high blood pressure and randomizes them to receive either Aprocitentan or Losartan for 24 months. After the study period, cardiovascular incidence in both groups is compared to determine which medication is superior. Which of the following would be the most appropriate measure of interest for this study?

A. Frequency of medication side effects in both groups

B. The average decrease in systolic blood pressure in each group

C. The average heart rate in participants receiving Drug A

D. The number of heart attacks in each group

E. The rate of patient adherence to the medication regimen

76. A prospective cohort study is designed to explore the relationship between vaper and the development of chronic obstructive pulmonary disease (COPD) in adults over the age of 40. One group in the study consists of adults who are current vapers and do not have COPD at baseline. Which of the following is the most appropriate comparison group for this study?

A. Adults who are current vapers and have COPD

B. Adults who are former vapers and do not have COPD

C. Adults who have never vaped and have COPD

D. Adults who have never vaped and do not have COPD

E. Adults who are former vapers and have COPD

77. A group of pediatric dermatologists plans to conduct a case-control study to evaluate the association between atopic dermatitis and seasonal allergies in children. The case group will consist of children who were diagnosed with atopic dermatitis by their pediatrician. Which of the following is the most appropriate control group for this study?

A. Children with a diagnosis of atopic dermatitis but no seasonal allergies

B. Children with a diagnosis of atopic dermatitis irrespective of seasonal allergy status

C. Children with no diagnosis of atopic dermatitis irrespective of seasonal allergy status

D. Children with no diagnosis of atopic dermatitis or seasonal allergies

   E. Children with a diagnosis of seasonal allergies but not atopic dermatitis

   F. Children with a diagnosis of seasonal allergies irrespective of atopic dermatitis status

78. A group of oncologists is planning a case-control study to explore the relationship between workplace chemical exposure and post-menopausal breast cancer. The case group consist of individuals diagnosed with breast cancer in the last 5 years. To ensure valid findings, they must select an appropriate control group for comparison. Which of the following is the most suitable control group?

   A. Post-menopausal women diagnosed with any type of cancer and a history of chemical exposure at work.

   B. Post-menopausal women diagnosed with breast cancer and a history of chemical exposure at work.

   C. Post-menopausal women diagnosed with breast cancer but without a history of chemical exposure at work.

   D. Post-menopausal women without a diagnosis of breast cancer and no history of chemical exposure at work.

   E. Post-menopausal women without a diagnosis of breast cancer but with a history of chemical exposure at work.

   F. Post-menopausal women without a diagnosis of breast cancer, regardless of their history of chemical exposure at work.

79. In a prospective cohort study investigating the link between physical inactivity and the risk of developing coronary artery disease (CAD), one group is composed of sedentary adults with no prior history of CAD at baseline. Researchers want to compare the incidence of CAD between physically inactive individuals and those who are active. Which of the following is the most appropriate comparison group for this study?

   A. Adults who are physically active and have CAD

   B. Adults who are physically active and do not have CAD

   C. Adults who are physically inactive and have CAD

   D. Adults who are moderately active and do not have CAD

   E. Adults with no history of CAD, regardless of activity level

80. Researchers are investigating a potential link between occupational exposure to asbestos and the development of lung cancer. They conduct a case-control study, where the case group consists of individuals diagnosed with lung cancer who have a history of asbestos exposure in the workplace. Which of the following populations should be selected as the control group?

    A. Individuals with lung cancer who have not been exposed to asbestos

    B. Individuals with lung cancer, regardless of asbestos exposure

    C. Individuals without lung cancer who have been exposed to asbestos

    D. Individuals without lung cancer who have not been exposed to asbestos

    E. Individuals without lung cancer, regardless of asbestos exposure

81. An increase in photoconjunctivitis cases has been reported among people living in a coastal region with high levels of sun exposure. A case-control study is designed to investigate the potential association between high sun exposure and the development of photoconjunctivitis. The case group includes individuals diagnosed with photoconjunctivitis who have a history of high sun exposure. Which of the following populations should be selected as the control group?

    A. Individuals without photoconjunctivitis who have high sun exposure

    B. Individuals without photoconjunctivitis who have low or no sun exposure

    C. Individuals without photoconjunctivitis, regardless of sun exposure

    D. Individuals with photoconjunctivitis who have low or no sun exposure

    E. Individuals with photoconjunctivitis, regardless of sun exposure

82. A group of orthopedic surgeons is planning a case-control study to investigate the potential association between anterior cruciate ligament (ACL) tears and the occurrence of patellar tendinitis in adolescent soccer players. The case group will consist of adolescent soccer players who have been diagnosed with an ACL tear during a routine examination. Which of the following is the most appropriate control group for this study?

    A. Adolescent non-soccer players with a diagnosis of ACL tear but not patellar tendinitis

B. Adolescent non-soccer players with a diagnosis of ACL tear irrespective of patellar tendinitis status

C. Adolescent soccer players with a diagnosis of ACL tear and patellar tendinitis

D. Adolescent soccer players with a diagnosis of ACL tear but not patellar tendinitis

E. Adolescent soccer players with a diagnosis of ACL tear irrespective of patellar tendinitis status

F. Adolescent soccer players with no diagnosis of ACL tear irrespective of patellar tendinitis status

G. Adolescent soccer players with no diagnosis of ACL tear or patellar tendinitis

83. Researchers are conducting a trial to assess the impact of a new behavioral therapy on reducing anxiety in patients with generalized anxiety disorder (GAD). A total of 200 participants are randomly assigned to either receive the therapy or be placed in a control group receiving standard care. What is the primary reason for using randomization in this trial?

A. To ensure both groups have an equal number of participants with varying levels of anxiety severity

B. To ensure that all participants are fully aware of the treatment they are receiving

C. To ensure the researchers can administer different therapies to each group

D. To ensure the researchers can observe the full effects of the new therapy on all participants

E. To ensure the study follows a predetermined sequence of participant enrollment

84. A clinical trial is set up to investigate the effect of imeglimin, a new diabetes drug on improving blood glucose levels in patients with type 2 diabetes. A total of 250 patients are recruited and randomly assigned to one of two groups: a treatment group receiving imeglimin and a control group receiving a placebo. Randomization in this study is to achieve which of the following?

    A. To allow both groups to be treated the same way, apart from the drug

    B. To allow the researchers to control for placebo effects across all patients

    C. To balance the distribution of confounding variables like age and disease duration between groups

    D. To ensure all participants have equal knowledge of the drug they receive

    E. To guarantee the drug is tested in a diverse group of patients

CHAPTER 5

85. A researcher is investigating the potential link between selective serotonin reuptake inhibitor (SSRI) use and the development of irritable bowel syndrome. He selects a group of individuals recently diagnosed with irritable bowel syndrome and a comparison group of healthy individuals with no history of irritable bowel syndrome. Both groups are then explored on their use of SSRI over the past 5 years. Which of the following measures of association is the researcher most likely to use in this study?

    A. Incidence rate

    B. Median survival

    C. Odds ratio

    D. Prevalence ratio

    E. Relative risk

86. A study aims to evaluate whether there is an association between childhood exposure to secondhand smoke and the development of asthma in adulthood. The researchers recruit adults with a current diagnosis of asthma and a control group of adults without asthma. Both groups are asked whether they were exposed to secondhand smoke during childhood. Which of the following statistical measures will most likely be used to quantify the association?

A. Attributable risk

B. Hazard ratio

C. Incidence density

D. Mean difference

E. Odds ratio

87. A clinical trial was conducted to evaluate the effectiveness of Wegovy in preventing heart attacks in obese patients. A group of obese patients was randomly assigned to receive either Wegovy or a placebo. Both groups were followed for 1 year to monitor the occurrence of heart attacks. What is the most appropriate measure of association the researchers are likely to use in this study?

A. Data table

B. Odds ratio

C. Prevalence

D. P-value

E. Relative risk

88. Researchers are studying the impact of a high-protein diet on the development of kidney disease in adults with diabetes. They selected a group of diabetic adults who consumed a high-protein diet and another group of diabetic adults who consumed a standard diet. Both groups were followed for 10 years to see how many developed kidney disease. Which measure of association is most appropriate for this cohort study?

A. Hazard ratio

B. Odds ratio

C. Prevalence ratio

D. P-value

E. Relative risk

89. A study investigates the relationship between the use of probiotics yogurt intake before and during pregnancy and the development of gestational diabetes mellitus (GDM) during 24-28 weeks of singleton pregnancy. The researchers found that 60 out of 140 high probiotic users developed GDM, while 70 out of 110 low probiotic users developed GDM. What is the odds of high probiotic intake in women with GDM compared to women with non GDM?

A. (40 / 110) / (80 / 140)

B. (40/ 120) / (70 × 130)

C. (40 × 60) / (80 × 70)

D. (60 × 110) / (70 × 140)

E. (60 × 140) / (70 × 110)

90. A clinical study is conducted to examine the association between aspirin use and the risk of stroke. Among 120 patients who regularly used aspirin, 15 experienced a stroke, while 25 out of 80 patients who did not use aspirin experienced a stroke. What is the odds ratio for stroke in aspirin users compared to non-users?

A. (15 / 120) / (25 / 80)

B. (15 × 105) / (25 × 65)

C. (15 × 55) / (25 × 105)

D. (15 × 65) / (25 × 105)

E. (15 × 80) / (25 × 105)

91. A team of researchers conducts a case-control study to determine whether herbal medication is associated with the development of liver cirrhosis in men aged 40-60. The data on herbal medication consumption for both cases (men with liver cirrhosis) and controls (men without liver cirrhosis) is presented below.

Herbal medication consumption	Liver Cirrhosis (+)	Liver Cirrhosis (-)	Total
High	65	40	105
Low	35	80	115
Total	100	120	220

What is the odds ratio of high alcohol consumption in men with liver cirrhosis compared to men without liver cirrhosis?

A. 0.50

B. 0.65

C. 2.03

D. 2.20

E. 3.71

92. A case-control study is conducted to investigate whether an excessive screen time is associated with the development of myopia in school-age children. Researchers collect data on the dietary habits of both cases (myopic children) and controls (normal vision, non-myopic children). The results are summarized below.

Excessive screen time	Myopia (+)	Myopia (-)	Total
Yes	180	120	300
No	90	150	240
Total	270	270	540

What is the estimated odds ratio for excessive screen time in myopic versus non-myopic children?

A. 0.5

B. 1.0

C. 1.5

D. 2.0

E. 2.5

93. A case-control study examines the relationship between high caffeine intake and anxiety disorders in adults. It includes 120 adults diagnosed with anxiety and 420 without. Data on caffeine consumption habit is collected, showing 30 with anxiety and 60 without reporting high caffeine intake. What is the estimated odds ratio of high caffeine intake for adults with anxiety compared to those without?

A. 0.67

B. 1.50

C. 1.67

D. 1.75

E. 2.00

94. A case-control study investigates the link between chronic sleep deprivation and the risk of depression in middle-aged adults. It includes 100 adults with depression and 440 without. The researchers assess sleep patterns in both groups. Among those with depression, 16 reported chronic sleep deprivation, compared to 20 in the non-depressed group. What is the estimated odds ratio of chronic sleep deprivation in adults with depression compared to those without?

   A. 2.67

   B. 3.52

   C. 4.00

   D. 6.80

   E. 8.00

95. A 50-year-old man visits the clinic concerned about his risk of developing coronary artery disease (CAD) because he has a family history of heart conditions. A recent cohort study looked at the risk of CAD in individuals based on their exercise habits. The study reported that, compared to individuals who exercise regularly, the relative risk (RR) of CAD in individuals who lead a sedentary lifestyle is 3.5, and the RR in those who exercise occasionally is 1.5. What is the relative risk of CAD for individuals with a sedentary lifestyle compared to those who exercise occasionally?

   A. 0.43

   B. 1.50

   C. 2.00

   D. 2.33

   E. 3.50

96. A 60-year-old woman comes in for her annual checkup and asks about the risk of osteoporosis as she ages. She is particularly concerned because her mother had osteoporosis. A cohort study assessed the relative risk of osteoporosis in women based on calcium intake. The study showed that, compared to women with high calcium intake, the relative risk (RR) of osteoporosis in women with low calcium intake is 2.8, and for those with moderate calcium intake, the RR is 1.6. Based on the study, what is the relative risk of osteoporosis for women with low calcium intake compared to those with moderate calcium intake?

A. 0.57

B. 1.00

C. 1.60

D. 1.75

E. 2.80

97. Evolocumab is a monoclonal antibody used as an immunotherapy medication for the treatment of hyperlipidemia. A study aimed to evaluate the impact of evolocumab on the risk of cardiovascular accidents (CVA). During a 7-year follow-up, 80 out of 1,000 participants who had taken evolocumab experienced a CVA, compared to 200 out of 2,000 participants who had not received evolocumab. What is the relative risk of developing CVA in participants who received evolocumab compared to those who received a placebo?

A. (80/200) / (920/1800)

B. (80/280) / (920×2720)

C. (80/1000) / (200/2000)

D. (80/200) - (920/1800)

E. (80/1000) - (200×2000)

98. A cohort study examined the role of statins in preventing stroke in patients with high cholesterol. Over a 6-year period, 70 out of 500 patients who were on statins developed a stroke, while 110 out of 400 patients who did not take statins experienced a stroke. What is the relative risk of developing a stroke in patients taking statins compared to those not taking statins?

A. (70×290)/(110×430)

B. (70×400)-(110×500)

C. (70/180)/(430/720)

D. (70/500)/(110/400)

E. (110/400)/(70/500)

99. A study was conducted to evaluate whether a new antibiotic prophylaxis could reduce the risk of hospital-acquired infections in post-surgical patients. The trial included 400 patients, randomly assigned to either receive the new antibiotic (200 patients) or a placebo (200 patients). Results showed that 10 patients in the antibiotic group developed a hospital-acquired infection, compared to 40 patients in the placebo group. What is the relative risk reduction (RRR) for hospital-acquired infections among patients who received the new antibiotic?

A. 0.05

B. 0.15

C. 0.20

D. 0.25

E. 0.75

100. Researchers conducted a study to evaluate the effectiveness of a new diet program aimed at preventing type 2 diabetes in individuals with prediabetes. The study enrolled 120 participants, 60 of whom followed the new diet program, while the other 60 followed standard care. After 3 years, 15 participants in the diet group developed diabetes, compared to 25 participants in the standard care group. What is the relative risk reduction (RRR) for developing diabetes in participants who followed the new diet program?

A. 0.050

B. 0.075

C. 0.125

D. 0.400

E. 0.600

101. A 40-year-old man visits his doctor for a regular checkup and expresses concern about his risk of developing cardiovascular disease (CVD), given his sedentary lifestyle. A recent cohort study followed 500 adults for 10 years, investigating the link between physical activity levels and CVD risk. The results are as follows:

lifestyle	Developed CVD	Did not develop CVD	Total
Sedentary	50	100	150
Physically active	40	310	350
Total	90	410	500

If this patient has low physical activity levels, what is his 10-year risk of developing cardiovascular disease?

A. 0.10

B. 0.11

C. 0.24

D. 0.33

E. 0.55

102. A 60-year-old man comes in for his annual checkup, concerned about his risk of developing lung cancer due to his history of smoking. A cohort study tracked 400 men over a 15-year period, evaluating their smoking habits and the risk of developing lung cancer. The study results are as follows:

Smoking habit	Developed lung cancer	Did not develop lung cancer	Total
Heavy smoker	40	60	100
Non-smoker	20	280	300
Total	60	340	400

Assuming the patient is a heavy smoker, what is his 15-year risk of developing lung cancer?

A. 0.07

B. 0.10

C. 0.17

D. 0.40

E. 0.67

103. Researchers conducted a trial to evaluate the impact of a new vaccine in reducing the incidence of pneumonia in elderly adults. A total of 800 participants, aged 65 and older, are randomly assigned to receive either the new vaccine (400 participants) or a placebo (400 participants). After 1 year, the following results are recorded:

Pneumonia Occurrence	Yes	No	Total
Vaccine	40	360	400
Placebo	60	340	400
Total	100	700	800

What is the absolute risk reduction (ARR) for pneumonia in patients who received the vaccine compared to those who received the placebo?

A. (40/400) - (60/400) = -0.05

B. (60/400) - (40/400) = 0.05

C. (60/400) / (40/400) = 1.5

D. (60/400) - (40/400) / (60/400) = 0.33

E. 1 / [(60/400) - (40/400)] = 20.0

104. A randomized trial evaluates whether a new chemotherapy drug reduces tumor recurrence in early-stage lung cancer. 300 patients are enrolled, with 150 assigned to the new drug and 150 to standard chemotherapy. After 2 years, the following data are reported:

Tumour Recurrence	Yes	No	Total
New drug	20	130	150
Standard	35	115	150
Total	55	245	300

What is the absolute risk reduction for tumour recurrence in patients treated with the new chemotherapy drug compared to standard chemotherapy?

A. (20/150) - (35/150) = -0.1

B. (35/150) - (20/150) = 0.1

C. (35/150) - (20/150) / (35/150) = 0.43

D. (35/150) / (20/150) = 1.75

E. 1 / [(35/150) - (20/150)] = 10.0

105. A clinical trial compared the side effects of a new antiemetic drug versus a placebo in preventing postoperative nausea in patients undergoing laparoscopic surgery. A total of 1,000 patients were randomized, with 500 patients receiving the new antiemetic and 500 receiving the placebo. The results showed 80 cases of nausea per 500 patients in the new antiemetic group and 60 cases per 500 patients in the placebo group. Which of the following is the best estimate of the absolute risk increase (ARI) for nausea in patients receiving the new antiemetic compared to placebo?

A.   (60/500) - (80/500)

B.   (80/500) - (60/500)

C.   (60/500) / (80/500)

D.   (80/500) / (60/500)

E.   1 / [(80/500) - (60/500)]

106. A randomized controlled trial studied the effects of a new sleep medication on the risk of falls in 800 elderly patients. The patients were randomized to receive either the new sleep medication (400 patients) or a placebo (400 patients). The primary outcome was the incidence of falls during the 6-month follow-up period. The results showed 90 cases of falls per 400 patients in the new sleep medication group and 60 cases per 400 patients in the placebo group. Which of the following is the best estimate of the absolute risk increase (ARI) for falls with the new sleep medication compared to placebo?

A.   (60/400) - (90/400)

B.   (90/400) - (60/400)

C.   (60/400) / (90/400)

D.   (90/400) / (60/400)

E.   1 / [(90/400) - (60/400)]

107. Researchers conducted a study to assess the efficacy of a new pneumonia vaccine in reducing the incidence of pneumonia in elderly adults aged 65 and older. After 3 years of follow-up, 95 of 100 participants who received the vaccine did not develop pneumonia, compared to 85 of 100 participants who did not receive the vaccine. Based on these results, which of the following represents the approximate number of patients who need to be vaccinated to prevent one additional case of pneumonia over 3 years?

A. 5

B. 10

C. 15

D. 20

E. 100

108. A randomized trial assessed whether adding a new antidepressant to standard therapy reduces recurrent of major depressive episodes. After 2 years, 92 of 100 patients on the new antidepressant regimen did not experience a depressive episode, compared to 85 of 100 patients on the standard therapy regimen alone. Which of the following represents the approximate number of patients who need to be treated with the new antidepressant to prevent one additional patient from experiencing a depressive episode within 2 years?

A. 2

B. 7

C. 8

D. 15

E. 19

109. Researchers conducted a 10-year study to assess the efficacy of a new colon cancer screening program in reducing the incidence of colon cancer in middle-aged adults. The study compared patients who underwent the new screening protocol to those who followed the standard screening protocol.

Colon cancer	Number of patients in new screening group	Number of patients in standard screening group
Present	8	16
Absent	992	984

Based on these results, how many patients need to undergo the new screening protocol to prevent one additional case of colon cancer?

A. 8

B. 75

C. 125

D. 200

E. 992

110. A study was conducted to evaluate the efficacy of a new prophylactic antibiotic, Antibiopro, in reducing the incidence of hospital-acquired infections (HAIs) in post-surgical patients. The study compared patients treated with Antibiopro to those treated with standard prophylactic antibiotics.

Hospital-acquired infection	Number of patients treated with Antibiopro	Number of patients treated with standard antibiotics
Infected	12	24
Not infected	988	976

Based on these results, how many patients need to be treated with Antibiopro to prevent one additional hospital-acquired infection?

A. 12

B. 24

C. 50

D. 83

E. 100

111. A clinical trial was conducted to assess the safety of a new broad-spectrum antibiotic for treating skin infections. The results of the trial showed that 8% of patients treated with the new antibiotic developed a rash, compared to 3% of patients treated with a standard antibiotic. Based on these results, how many patients need to be treated with the new antibiotic to cause one additional case of rash?

A. 5

B. 20

C. 33

D. 50

E. 125

112. A double-blind placebo-controlled trial was conducted to evaluate the safety profile of a new antidepressant in adults with major depressive disorder. The study reported that 9% of patients treated with the new antidepressant experienced insomnia, compared to 4% of patients receiving a placebo. Based on these results, how many patients need to be treated with the new antidepressant to cause one additional case of insomnia?

A. 4

B. 5

C. 9

D. 20

E. 25

113. A study was conducted to assess the safety of a new antiviral drug for treating hepatitis C. The study examined the incidence of liver toxicity in patients treated with the new drug versus those receiving standard antiviral therapy. The results are shown below:

Liver toxicity	New antiviral drug	Standard therapy
Yes	15	5
No	285	295

Based on these results, which of the following best represents the number needed to harm (NNH) for the new antiviral drug?

A. 5

B. 15

C. 20

D. 30

E. 50

114. A pharmaceutical company evaluates the safety of a new oral contraceptive, focusing on the risk of thrombosis. The study compares the incidence of thrombosis in women using the new contraceptive to those using an older, well-established oral contraceptive. The results are as follows:

	New contraceptive	Older contraceptive
Thrombosis cases	12	4
No thrombosis	488	496

Based on these results, which of the following best represents the number needed to harm (NNH) for the new oral contraceptive?

A. 4

B. 8

C. 12

D. 16

E. 63

115. A large retrospective cohort study examines the link between excessive alcohol consumption and liver cirrhosis in a population of European men. Over a 12-year period, those with heavy alcohol use have 4.5 times the risk of developing cirrhosis compared to those who do not drink excessively (relative risk = 4.5, 95% confidence interval = 3.1-6.0). Based on this study, what percentage of liver cirrhosis cases in heavy drinkers can be attributed to excessive alcohol consumption?

A. 35%

B. 50%

C. 65%

D. 77%

E. 85%

116. A case-control study is conducted to evaluate the relationship between a sedentary lifestyle and type 2 diabetes among adults. Results show that adults with a sedentary lifestyle have 2.8 times the risk of developing type 2 diabetes compared to active individuals (relative risk = 2.8, 95% confidence interval = 2.0-3.6). According to the study findings, what percentage of type 2 diabetes cases in sedentary adults can be attributed to a sedentary lifestyle?

A. 29%

B. 50%

C. 64%

D. 71%

E. 80%

117. A clinical trial is conducted to test the efficacy of a new antiviral drug, AVX, in reducing the recurrence of viral hepatitis after liver transplantation. The recurrence rate of viral hepatitis in the standard therapy group is 10%. Regulatory authorities will approve AVX if it reduces the recurrence rate by at least 50% compared to standard therapy. What is the maximal acceptable recurrence rate for patients treated with AVX plus standard therapy?

    A. 2%

    B. 3%

    C. 4%

    D. 5%

    E. 6%

118. A new anticoagulant, Drug X, is being tested in a study to determine its efficacy in reducing the incidence of recurrent deep vein thrombosis (DVT) compared to standard therapy. The current recurrence rate of DVT in the standard therapy group is 6%. Drug X will be approved if it reduces the incidence of recurrent DVT by at least 33%. What is the maximal incidence of recurrent DVT acceptable for patients treated with Drug X?

    A. 1%

    B. 2%

    C. 3%

    D. 4%

    E. 5%

119. Researchers conduct a study to determine whether a new influenza vaccine reduces the incidence of flu in elderly individuals aged 65 and older. Participants are randomly assigned to receive either the new vaccine or a placebo before the flu season begins. At the end of the flu season, the incidence of laboratory-confirmed influenza is compared between the two groups. The relative risk of developing influenza among those receiving the new vaccine compared to the placebo group is 0.50 (95% confidence interval of (0.35–0.72). Which of the following is the most appropriate conclusion about the effect of the vaccine on the risk of influenza?

    A. Receiving the vaccine reduces the risk of influenza by 50%

    B. The risk of developing influenza in the vaccine group is 0.5%

   C.   The risk of developing influenza is reduced by 50% with the vaccine

   D.   The vaccine has no significant effect on the risk of influenza

   E.   The vaccine increases the risk of developing influenza by 50%

120. A group of researchers studies the effect of a structured weight-loss program on the incidence of obesity in overweight individuals over a 2-year period. Participants are randomly assigned to either the weight-loss program or a standard care group that receives general dietary advice. The incidence of obesity, defined as a body mass index (BMI) ≥ 30, is recorded at the end of the study. The relative risk of obesity in the weight-loss program group compared to the standard care group is 0.65 (95% confidence interval of 0.48–0.88). Which of the following is the most appropriate conclusion about the effect of the weight-loss program on obesity risk?

   A.   The risk of developing obesity in the weight-loss group is 0.65%

   B.   The risk of developing obesity is reduced by 35% in the weight-loss program

   C.   The weight-loss program has no significant effect on obesity risk

   D.   The weight-loss program increases the risk of obesity by 35%

   E.   The weight-loss program reduces the risk of obesity by 65%

121. Researchers conducted a clinical trial to compare the effectiveness of two cholesterol-lowering drugs, Drug A and Drug B, in preventing heart attacks. The absolute risk reduction (ARR) of Drug A compared to placebo was 0.07, while the ARR of Drug B compared to placebo was 0.15. Based on these results, which of the following statements best describes the comparison of Drugs A and B?

   A.   Drug A requires treating fewer patients to prevent 1 additional heart attack compared to Drug B, so Drug A is more effective

   B.   Drug A requires treating more patients to prevent 1 additional heart attack compared to Drug B, so Drug A is less effective

   C.   Drug A and Drug B require treating the same number of patients to prevent 1 additional heart attack, so they are equally effective

   D.   Drug B requires treating more patients to prevent 1 additional heart attack compared to Drug A, so Drug B is less effective

   E.   Drug B requires treating fewer patients to prevent 1 additional heart attack compared to Drug A, so Drug B is more effective

122. A clinical trial evaluates the risk of serious adverse effects from two antibiotics, Drug C and Drug D, used to treat bacterial pneumonia. The absolute risk increase (ARI) for adverse effects of Drug C compared to placebo is 0.04, while the ARI for Drug D compared to placebo is 0.10. Which of the following is the most appropriate conclusion regarding the risk of adverse effects from Drugs C and D?

   A. Drug C requires treating fewer patients to cause 1 additional adverse effect compared to Drug D, so Drug C is more harmful

   B. Drug C requires treating more patients to cause 1 additional adverse effect compared to Drug D, so Drug C is less harmful

   C. Drug C and Drug D require treating the same number of patients to cause 1 additional adverse effect, so they are equally harmful

   D. Drug D requires treating more patients to cause 1 additional adverse effect compared to Drug C, so Drug D is less harmful

   E. Drug D requires treating fewer patients to cause 1 additional adverse effect compared to Drug C, so Drug D is more harmful

123. A study was conducted to assess the efficacy of two new pain relievers, Drug E and Drug F, for reducing chronic back pain. The absolute risk reduction (ARR) for Drug E compared to placebo was 0.08, and the ARR for Drug F compared to placebo was 0.20. Which of the following statements comparing the effectiveness of Drugs E and F is most appropriate?

   A. Drug E requires treating more patients to achieve pain relief in 1 additional person compared to Drug F, so Drug E is less effective

   B. Drug E requires treating fewer patients to achieve pain relief in 1 additional person compared to Drug F, so Drug E is more effective

   C. Drug E and Drug F require treating the same number of patients to achieve pain relief in 1 additional person, so they are equally effective

   D. Drug F requires treating more patients to achieve pain relief in 1 additional person compared to Drug E, so Drug F is less effective

   E. Drug F requires treating fewer patients to achieve pain relief in 1 additional person compared to Drug E, so Drug F is more effective

CHAPTER 6

124. A group of researchers conducts a case-control study to evaluate the risk factors associated with acute myocardial infarction in elderly men. They enrol 100 men who have had a recent AMI and 200 age-matched controls who have not. The frequency of risk factors, such as smoking, hypertension, and high cholesterol levels, is compared between the two groups. Which of the following is the most appropriate null hypothesis for this study?

   A. Hazard ratio is equal to 1

   B. Hazard ratio is not equal to 1

   C. Odds ratio is equal to 1

   D. Odds ratio is not equal to 1

   E. Relative risk is equal to 1

   F. Relative risk is not equal to 1

125. Researchers are conducting a prospective cohort study to assess the relationship between regular physical activity and the development of Alzheimer's disease among older adults. They follow 1,000 participants over 10 years, comparing the incidence of Alzheimer's between those who engage in regular physical activity and those who do not. Which of the following is the most appropriate null hypothesis for this study?

   A. Hazard ratio is equal to 1

   B. Hazard ratio is not equal to 1

   C. Odds ratio is equal to 1

   D. Odds ratio is not equal to 1

   E. Relative risk is equal to 1

   F. Relative risk is not equal to 1

126. A team of researchers is conducting a trial to test the effectiveness of Talquetamab, a humanized monoclonal antibody used in the treatment of multiple myeloma. They find that their sample size is too small, resulting in inconclusive findings regarding the therapy's efficacy. To enhance their ability to detect a true effect if one exists, what should they prioritize in their study design?

    A. α

    B. $1 - \beta$

    C. Type I error

    D. Type II error

    E. Selection bias

127. In a study assessing the effects of carnitine which increases fatty acid oxidation, as a dietary supplement on weight loss, researchers determine that the mean weight loss after 12 weeks is 8 kg in the supplement group and 5 kg in the placebo group. The probability that this observed difference is due to random chance is reported as 4%. Additionally, there is a 10% probability of concluding that there is no difference in weight loss when there is one in reality. What is the power of the study?

    A. 0.04

    B. 0.60

    C. 0.90

    D. 0.94

    E. 0.96

128. A randomized controlled trial investigates the impact of a new educational program on improving patient adherence to medication. The study reports that adherence rates are 75% in the group receiving the educational program compared to 60% in the control group. The p-value for the difference in adherence rates is found to be 0.02, and 80% chance of concluding that there is difference when there actually is none. What is the power of the study?

    A. 0.02

    B. 0.20

C.   0.60

D.   0.75

E.   0.80

129. A study examines the effects of dietary fibre intake on blood glucose levels among prediabetes. The authors conclude, "The analysis indicates a strong negative correlation (r = -0.70) between fibre intake and blood glucose levels, with a probability of observing this result due to by chance is 4%, and 75% chance of rejecting the null hypothesis when it is false." Based on this conclusion, which of the following represents the p-value and the power of the correlation test in the study?

A.   p-value of 0.04; power of 0.75

B.   p-value of 0.04; power of 0.80

C.   p-value of 0.05; power of 0.80

D.   p-value of 0.05; power of 0.90

E.   p-value of 0.25; power of 0.75

F.   p-value of 0.25; power of 0.60

130. A study investigates the relationship between physical activity levels and cholesterol levels in middle-aged adults. The researchers report the following findings: "Our analysis reveals a negative correlation between physical activity and cholesterol levels (r = -0.9). The likelihood of observing this result due to random chance is 2%, with a 15% chance of concluding no relationship between the physical activity levels and cholesterol levels when one truly exists." Which of the following most accurately represents the p-value and the power of the correlation test in the study?

A.   p-value of 0.02; power of 0.80

B.   p-value of 0.02; power of 0.85

C.   p-value of 0.02; power of 0.90

D.   p-value of 0.05; power of 0.80

E.   p-value of 0.05; power of 0.85

F.   p-value of 0.05; power of 0.90

131. A randomized controlled trial tests the antihypertensive treatment effect of a quadruple single-pill combination in hypertensive patients. The researchers set the alpha level at 0.05. After preliminary analysis, they find promising results and decide to lower the alpha level to 0.01 for the final analysis. What impact will this change likely have on the study's results?

    A. More findings will be reported as significant

    B. The criteria for claiming a statistically significant effect will become more stringent

    C. The power of the study will significantly increase

    D. The probability of Type I errors will increase

    E. The sample size will be reduced

132. In a study assessing the impact of a new educational program on patient outcomes in a healthcare setting, researchers choose an alpha value of 0.05 to determine statistical significance. After conducting the analysis, they find a p-value of 0.04. If the alpha level had been set at 0.01 instead, what would have been the result regarding this finding?

    A. The findings would indicate a stronger treatment effect

    B. The findings would likely lead to a Type I error

    C. The result would be considered significant at the 0.01 level

    D. The result would not be considered statistically significant

    E. The result would still be considered significant

133. A researcher conducts a study on gender differences in self-reported symptoms of depression among patients with acute coronary syndrome. Somatic depressive symptoms were measured using BDI-II question 16 (sleep disturbance), question 18 (appetite disturbance), and question 20 (fatigue). A patient was identified as positive for somatic depressive symptoms if the patient rated all three items as 1 or above. If a patient rated 0 on any of the three items, he or she was categorized as negative for somatic depressive symptoms. The presence of somatic depressive symptoms is compared across genders.

Gender	Somatic depressive symptoms		Total
	Present	Absent	
Male	12	529	541
Female	19	229	248
Total	31	758	789

Which of the following is the best statistical method to estimate the association between exercise frequency and obesity status in this study?

A. Analysis of variance

B. Chi-square test

C. Correlational analysis

D. Meta-analysis

E. Two-sample t-test

134. Using the Korean Genome and Epidemiology Study (KoGES-8), the researchers explored the prediction factors for diabetes, one of the physical factors of interest is weight gain or weight loss in the past month. Participants are classified based on their weight (weight gain vs. weight loss) and diabetes status (diabetic vs. non-diabetic). The data collected is displayed in the following table:

Disease condition		Not have diabetes	Have diabetes	Total
Weight	Gain	2329	491	2820
	Loss	263	83	346
Total		2592	574	3166

Which statistical test is most appropriate for determining the association between weight and diabetes status in this study?

A. Analysis of variance

B. Chi-square test

C. Correlational analysis

D. Meta-analysis

E. Two-sample t-test

135. Researchers are studying the effect of a flexitarian diet on weight loss. In a controlled trial, Group A (participants on the flexitarian diet) loses an average of 8.2 pounds with a standard deviation of 2.5 pounds, while Group B (participants on a standard diet) loses an average of 5.7 pounds with a standard deviation of 3.0 pounds. Which statistical test should the researchers use to compare the weight loss between these two groups?

    A. ANOVA

    B. Chi-square test

    C. Correlation analysis

    D. Regression analysis

    E. Two-sample t-test

136. A nutrition study measures cholesterol levels in two different populations. Population A has a mean cholesterol level of 190 mg/dL with a standard deviation of 15 mg/dL, while Population B has a mean cholesterol level of 205 mg/dL with a standard deviation of 20 mg/dL. To determine if there is a significant difference in cholesterol levels between these two populations, which statistical method should be employed?

    A. ANOVA

    B. Chi-square test

    C. Paired t-test

    D. Regression analysis

    E. Two-sample t-test

137. Researchers are investigating the impact of multidisciplinary vocational rehabilitation program with an integrated work and lifestyle intervention included 4 weeks of inpatient stay followed-up by 5 meetings on a weight loss program on participants' body mass index (BMI). They measure the BMI ot the participants before the program begins (mean 30.2, standard deviation 2.3) and after three months of participation (mean 28.5, standard deviation of 2.0). Which statistical test is most appropriate for comparing the BMI measurements before and after the program?

    A. ANOVA

    B. Chi-square test

    C. Correlation analysis

    D.   Paired t-test

    E.   Two-sample t-test

138. A research study is conducted to assess the effectiveness of a smoking cessation program. Participants' carbon monoxide levels are measured before the program starts and again after they have completed the program. The average carbon monoxide level before the program is found to be 12.5 ppm with a standard deviation of 1.5, while the average level after the program is 6.8 ppm with a standard deviation of 1.2. Which statistical test should the researchers use to compare the carbon monoxide levels before and after the cessation program?

    A.   Analysis of variance

    B.   Chi-square test

    C.   Paired t-test

    D.   Regression analysis

    E.   Two-sample t-test

139. A researcher is interested in the effect of three types of exercise programs (aerobic, strength training, and flexibility training) on participants' cardiovascular fitness levels, measured by VO_2 max. Each program includes 30 participants, and their VO_2 max is measured after a 12-week intervention. What is the most suitable statistical analysis to determine if there are significant differences in VO_2 max among the three exercise groups?

    A.   Analysis of variance

    B.   Chi-square test

    C.   Independent t-test

    D.   Kruskal-Wallis test

    E.   Regression analysis

140. A clinical trial is conducted to assess the effectiveness of four different antihypertensive medications on blood pressure reduction. Each medication is administered to a group of 40 patients, and their blood pressure is measured before and after treatment. To compare the average blood pressure reduction across the four medication groups, which statistical method should be used?

   A. Analysis of variance

   B. Logistic regression

   C. Mann-Whitney U test

   D. Pearson correlation coefficient

   E. Two-sample t-test

141. A research team investigates the effect of different diets on weight loss among participants over a 12-week program. Participants are divided into three groups: Group A follows a low-carb diet, Group B follows a Mediterranean diet, and Group C follows a low-fat diet. At the end of the study, the researchers want to compare the mean weight loss among all three groups. Which statistical test is most appropriate for this analysis?

   A. Analysis of variance

   B. Chi-square test

   C. Independent t-test

   D. Paired t-test

   E. Regression analysis

142. A study evaluates the impact of three exercise regimens on cardiovascular fitness in older adults: Group I (aerobic exercise), Group II (resistance training), and Group III (combined both aerobic and resistance training). After 8 weeks, VO_2 max improvements are measured. Which statistical method is used to determine if there are significant differences among the three groups?

   A. ANOVA

   B. Chi-square test

   C. Correlation analysis

   D. Independent t-test

   E. Paired t-test

143. A clinical trial assesses the effectiveness of three different antihypertensive medications for hypertension in pregnancy. Patients are assigned to one of three treatment groups: Group A receives diazoxide, Group B receives nicardipine, and Group C receives hydralazine. The researchers want to compare time taken for achieving the target BP across the three groups. Which statistical test is appropriate for this comparison?

    A. Analysis of variance

    B. Chi-square test

    C. Logistic regression

    D. Paired t-test

    E. Two-sample t-test

144. A health economist is studying the factors that influence healthcare costs in patients with chronic diseases. They plan to include variables such as age, BMI, number of medications, and exercise frequency in their analysis. To evaluate how these factors predict total healthcare costs, which statistical method is most appropriate?

    A. Analysis of variance

    B. Chi-square test

    C. Odds ratio

    D. Regression analysis

    E. T-test

145. A diabetes research team is examining how dietary fibre intake and physical activity levels affect fasting blood glucose levels in adults with type 2 diabetes. The study gathers data on fibre intake (grams/day), weekly physical activity (minutes/week), and fasting blood glucose (mg/dL), while adjusting for medication use and duration of diabetes. Which statistical technique is best suited to determine the relationship between dietary fibre intake, physical activity, and fasting blood glucose levels, considering medication use and diabetes duration?

    A. Analysis of variance

    B. Chi-square test

    C. Meta-analysis

    D. Paired t-test

    E. Regression analysis

146. A psychologist is studying the relationship between quality of sleep and cognitive performance in college students. Based on Insomnia Severity Index (ISI) scores, which can be between 0-28, sleep quality was assessed. ISI values range from 0-28. Montreal Cognitive Assessment (MoCA) score ranging from 0-30 was used to determine the cognitive performance. To analyse whether there is a relationship between sleep quality and cognitive performance scores, which statistical test is most appropriate?

A. Analysis of variance

B. Chi-square test

C. Correlation analysis

D. Independent t-test

E. Regression analysis

147. In a study involving 250 patients, the relationship between the number of cigarettes smoked per day (continuous variable) and forced expiratory volume (FEV1) in litres (continuous variable) is being analysed. The researcher wants to determine if there is a linear relationship between these two variables. Which statistical method should be used to assess the strength and direction of this relationship?

A. Chi-square test

B. Linear regression

C. Paired t-test

D. Pearson correlation

E. Spearman's rank correlation

148. A nutritionist is studying the relationship between fruit and vegetable intake and body mass index (BMI) among a group of 300 adults. The researcher finds that as fruit and vegetable intake increases, BMI tends to decrease, with a strong correlation between the two variables. According to this, which of the following statements best describes the associated correlation coefficient?

A. It is negative and probably closer to 0 than to -1

B. It is negative and probably closer to -1 than to 0

C. It is positive and probably closer to 0 than to 1

D. It is positive and probably closer to 1 than to 0

149. A psychologist conducts a study to assess the relationship between hours of sleep and levels of anxiety in a sample of 150 college students. The analysis reveals that lower levels of sleep are associated with higher anxiety levels. The correlation coefficient calculated from the data is weak. Based on this information, which of the following statements best describes the associated correlation coefficient?

A. It is negative and probably closer to 0 than to -1

B. It is negative and probably closer to -1 than to 0

C. It is positive and probably closer to 0 than to 1

D. It is positive and probably closer to 1 than to 0

150. Inflammatory markers are useful in many clinical settings, including tracking disease activity in conditions like systemic lupus erythematosus (SLE). A new marker is being studied in patients with active SLE flares. As the level of this marker in the blood (mg/L) increases, the C-reactive protein (CRP) level decreases. The correlation analysis is strong and significant relationship. Based on this, which statement best describes the correlation coefficient?

A. It is negative and probably closer to 0 than to -1

B. It is negative and probably closer to -1 than to 0

C. It is positive and probably closer to 0 than to 1

D. It is positive and probably closer to 1 than to 0

151. Serum cholesterol levels and systolic blood pressure are commonly measured in patients at risk for cardiovascular disease. A new study investigates the relationship between these two variables in a cohort of 200 patients with hypertension. Serum cholesterol (in mg/dL) and systolic blood pressure (in mmHg) are plotted for each patient, and the following scatterplot is generated.

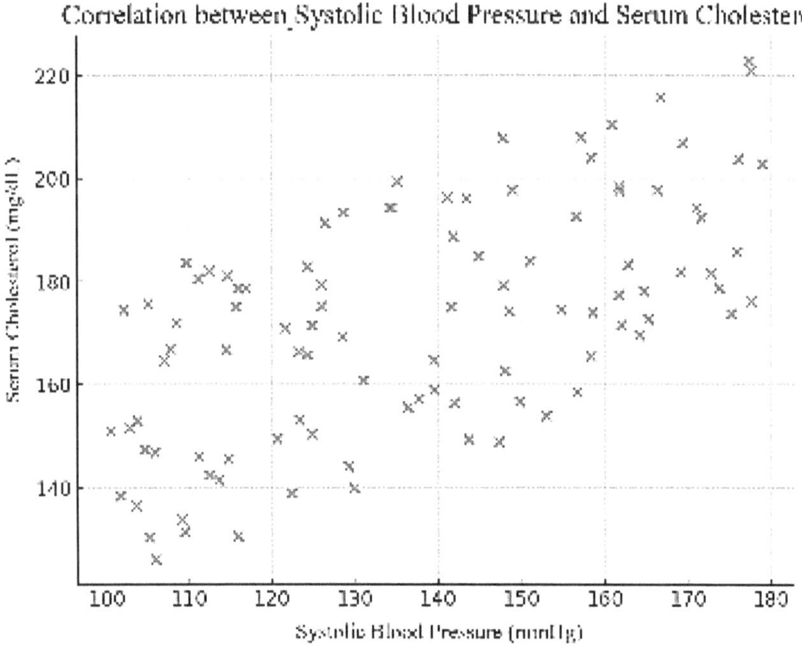

Based on the plot, the correlation coefficient between the two variables is most likely closest to which of the following values?

A. -0.7

B. -0.4

C. 0

D. +0.2

E. +0.6

152. Cortisol levels are clinically useful in assessing adrenal gland activity, especially in conditions like Addison's disease or Cushing's syndrome. A new adrenal function test (nmol/L) is being investigated to track adrenal activity during different stress responses. When the serum cortisol (µg/dL) is plotted against the new adrenal function test (nmol/L), the following plot is obtained.

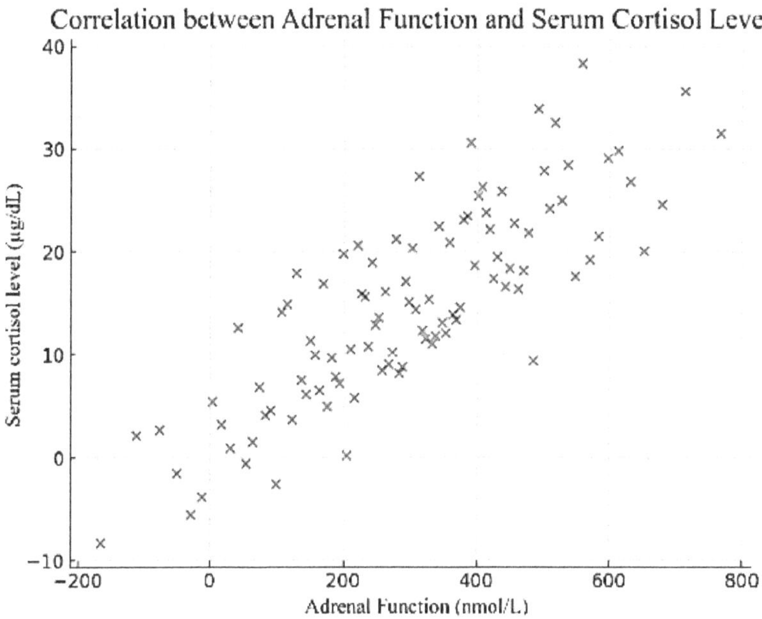

Based on the plot, the correlation coefficient between the two variables is closest to which of the following values?

A. +0.8

B. +0.3

C. 0

D. -0.3

E. -0.8

153. Researchers are investigating the correlation between physical activity levels (minutes of exercise per week) and cholesterol levels (mg/dL) in adults aged 30-50. They find a correlation coefficient of $r = -0.42$ ($p < 0.05$) between physical activity and cholesterol levels. Which of the following interpretations is most accurate?

    A. Increased cholesterol levels significantly reduce physical activity among adults.

    B. Increased physical activity leads to a significant decrease in cholesterol levels in adults.

    C. There is a statistically significant negative linear relationship between physical activity and cholesterol levels.

    D. There is a statistically significant positive linear relationship between physical activity and cholesterol levels.

    E. There is no significant relationship between physical activity and cholesterol levels.

154. A medical study is conducted to assess the relationship between dietary sodium intake (mg/day) and blood pressure (mmHg) among adults. The researchers report a correlation coefficient of $r = 0.55$ ($p < 0.01$) between sodium intake and systolic blood pressure. What is the most accurate interpretation of these findings?

    A. Decreased sodium intake significantly lowers systolic blood pressure.

    B. Increased sodium intake causes a statistically significant decrease in blood pressure.

    C. Sodium intake has no impact on blood pressure in adults.

    D. There is a statistically significant negative linear relationship between sodium intake and blood pressure.

    E. There is a statistically significant positive linear relationship between sodium intake and blood pressure.

155. In a study examining the impact of a intermittent fasting intervention on body mass index (BMI) in obese adults, researchers found a mean reduction in BMI of 2.5 kg/m² with a 95% confidence interval of -0.1 – 5.1 kg/m². Which of the following p-values would be most consistent with these findings?

    A. 0.02

    B. 0.04

    C. 0.06

    D. 0.12

    E. 0.25

156. A cohort study investigates the association between chronic exposure to high-decibel occupational noise and the risk of developing early-onset hearing loss. The hazard ratio for workers exposed to noise levels above 85 dB compared to those in quieter environments is reported as 2.7, with a 95% confidence interval of 1.8–4.3. Which of the following p-values is most likely?

    A. 0.02

    B. 0.07

    C. 0.10

    D. 0.15

    E. 0.50

157. A study was conducted to evaluate the effect of a new cognitive behaviour therapy (CBT) intervention on reducing obesity rates among children aged 6-12. After implementing the intervention, researchers found that the average weight loss in the intervention group was 5 kg, with a 95% confidence interval of 2-8 kg compared to the control group. Which of the following statements most accurately represents the impact of the educational intervention?

    A. The intervention causes weight gain

    B. The intervention has a significant effect on reducing weight

    C. The intervention is ineffective in reducing weight

    D. The intervention's effect is clinically irrelevant

    E. There is no evidence to suggest the intervention's effectiveness

158. In a double-blind, placebo-controlled trial on the antihypertensive treatment effect of a quadruple single-pill combination, researchers reported the between-group difference in systolic blood pressure was -4.6 mmHg with a 95% confidence interval of −9.7 to 0.6 mmHg. Which of the following statements best represents the results of this trial?

    A. The difference is not statistically significant

    B. The drug effect is clinically irrelevant

    C. The drug has no effect on blood pressure.

    D. The drug increases blood pressure

    E. The drug significantly lowers blood pressure

159. A clinical trial assessed the effects of a new weight loss drug on body mass index (BMI) over 12 weeks. The mean difference in BMI between the drug group and the placebo group was reported as follows:

Study	Mean BMI$_{Drug Group}$ − Mean BMI$_{Control Group}$ (kg/m^2) [95% CI]
1	-3.0 [-4.5, -1.5]
2	-0.2 [-1.8, 1.4]
3	-2.5 [-3.2, -1.0]
4	-0.8 [-1.6, -0.1]
5	-1.5 [-2.3, -0.7]
6	-0.6 [-0.8, -0.4]
Total	-1.4 [-2.1, -0.7]

Based on the analysis, what can be concluded?

A. A higher mean BMI was observed in the drug group overall.

B. The weight loss drug should be recommended for weight management.

C. The weight loss drug was associated with a statistically significant decrease in BMI.

D. All studies showed a statistically significant decrease in BMI.

E. There was no statistically significant change in BMI overall.

160. In a recent meta-analysis examining the effects of mindfulness meditation on anxiety levels, the following results were found:

Study	Mean Anxiety Reduction in Meditation Group - Control Group [95% CI]
1	-6.0 [-8.1, -3.9]
2	-0.5 [-2.5, 3.5]
3	-4.0 [-5.7, -2.3]
4	-2.5 [-4.0, -1.0]
5	-1.0 [-3.5, 1.5]
6	-1.5 [-1.0, 4.0]
Total	-2.8 [-3.4, -2.2]

Based on these findings, which of the following conclusions is most accurate?

A. All studies demonstrated a statistically significant reduction in anxiety levels.

B. Mindfulness meditation resulted in a higher mean anxiety level overall.

C. Mindfulness meditation should be recommended for anxiety management.

D. Mindfulness meditation was associated with a statistically significant reduction in anxiety levels.

E. There was no statistically significant change in anxiety levels overall.

161. A study is conducted to compare the effects of daily meditation versus no meditation on stress levels in university students. A total of 180 students are enrolled and randomly assigned in a 1:1 ratio to either the daily meditation group or the control group (no meditation). After 3 months, the meditation group shows a greater reduction in stress levels compared to the control group, with a mean difference in stress reduction of -5 points on a standardized scale (p = 0.04, predetermined significance level = 0.05). Which of the following is the most accurate interpretation of the results of this study?

A. The observed mean difference in stress reduction of -5 points is not statistically significant

B. The probability of observing a mean difference in stress reduction of -5 points is 0.04

C. There is a 4% chance of observing a mean difference in stress reduction of at least -5 points when no difference between groups is assumed

D. There is a 4% chance that a student practicing daily meditation will have a stress reduction of at least -5 points after 3 months

E. There is a 4% chance that the mean difference in stress reduction is biased in favour of the meditation group

162. Researchers investigate the effect of a moderate exercise program versus no exercise on sleep quality in adults with insomnia. A total of 250 adults are randomly assigned in a 1:1 ratio to either a moderate exercise group or a no-exercise control group. After 6 months, the exercise group shows an improvement in sleep quality compared to the control group, with a mean difference in sleep quality score of +4 points ($p = 0.02$, predetermined significance level $= 0.05$). Which of the following is the most accurate interpretation of the results of this study?

A. An adult in the moderate exercise group has a 2% chance of improving their sleep quality score by at least +4 points after 6 months

B. The mean difference of +4 points in sleep quality score is not statistically significant.

C. The likelihood of observing a +4 point mean difference in sleep quality score is 0.02.

D. The probability that the mean difference in sleep quality is biased toward the moderate exercise group is 2%.

E. There is a 2% probability of seeing a mean difference of at least +4 points in sleep quality when assuming no difference between the groups.

CHAPTER 7

163. A 50-year-old man with a history of high cholesterol is undergoing testing for lipid levels. The total cholesterol test is repeated three times using the same sample, and the results are 210 mg/dL, 215 mg/dL, and 220 mg/dL. Despite the variations in the results, they are all within a similar range. However, the true cholesterol level is known to be 180 mg/dL. Which of the following parameters is most likely to be low based on these test results?

   A. Accuracy

   B. Precision

   C. Sensitivity

   D. Specificity

   E. Validity

164. During the evaluation of a new hemoglobin A1c test device, three measurements of the same sample yield results of 5.5%, 5.6%, and 5.6%. Which of the following parameters is likely to be high with the new hemoglobin A1c test device?

   A. Accuracy

   B. Precision

   C. Sensitivity

   D. Specificity

   E. Validity

165. A research team is testing a new blood pressure monitor designed for home use. They measure a patient's blood pressure three times with the device, resulting in readings of 130/85 mmHg, 131/84 mmHg, and 129/86 mmHg. However, a standard sphygmomanometer measurement shows the true blood pressure to be 150/95 mmHg. Which of the following descriptions best characterizes the new blood pressure monitor?

   A. High accuracy; high precision

   B. High accuracy; low precision

C. High sensitivity; low specificity

D. Low accuracy; high precision

E. Low accuracy; low precision

F. Low sensitivity; high specificity

166. A new glucose monitoring device is tested for its reliability. In a series of tests, the device gives readings of 85 mg/dL, 96 mg/dL, and 134 mg/dL for a single patient sample. However, the laboratory reference measurement for the same sample indicates a glucose level of 130 mg/dL. Which of the following descriptions best characterizes the glucose monitoring device?

A. High accuracy; high precision

B. High accuracy; low precision

C. High sensitivity; low specificity

D. Low accuracy; high precision

E. Low accuracy; low precision

F. Low sensitivity; high specificity

167. A research team is assessing D-dimer as a diagnostic tool for deep vein thrombosis (DVT). The test is compared to duplex ultrasonography, the gold standard for DVT diagnosis. In a sample of 200 patients, 50 are confirmed to have DVT. The test shows a sensitivity of 90% and a specificity of 80%. How many false positives are present in the study?

A. 10

B. 20

C. 30

D. 40

E. 50

168. A clinical trial tests low-frequency electromagnetic waves for detecting early-stage breast cancer, comparing it to mammography (the gold standard). Out of 400 participants, 200 are diagnosed with breast cancer. The new test has a sensitivity of 95% and a specificity of 90%. How many false positives are in the study?

A. 10

B. 20

C. 30

D. 40

E. 50

169. A clinical trial is assessing protein dopa decarboxylase (DCC) for diagnosing Parkinson's disease. The sensitivity of the test is estimated at 80%, and the specificity at 90%. The trial includes 400 patients, of whom 100 are confirmed cases of Parkinson's disease based on the reference standard. What is the expected number of false negatives in this study?

A. 10

B. 20

C. 30

D. 40

E. 90

170. E-nose, a diagnostic test, detects volatile organic compounds (VOCs) in a person's breath, which are emitted by cancer cells. In a study assessing the test's effectiveness for diagnosing lung cancer, 200 patients with confirmed lung cancer and 100 without lung cancer were tested. The test demonstrated a sensitivity of 86% and a specificity of 95%. Based on these results, how many false negatives occurred in the study?

A. 5

B. 10

C. 14

D. 15

E. 28

171. The table below provides the results of a study investigating a new diagnostic test for tuberculosis (TB).

	TB present	No TB
Test positive	65	15
Test negative	35	85

What is the sensitivity of the new diagnostic test?

A. 19%

B. 29%

C. 65%

D. 71%

E. 81%

F. 85%

172. The study results for a new test diagnosing Lyme disease are shown in the table below.

New Diagnostic Test	Lyme Disease present	No Lyme Disease
Test positive	85	35
Test negative	15	165

What is the sensitivity of the new diagnostic test?

A. 29.1%

B. 70.9%

C. 82.5%

D. 85.0%

E. 91.7%

173. A clinical trial is conducted to assess a new test for diagnosing influenza. The comparison gold standard is viral culture. The study results are shown below:

Influenza Test	Positive viral culture	Negative viral culture
Test positive	90	30
Test negative	60	120

What is the specificity of the new test?

A. 33%

B. 60%

C. 67.7%

D. 75%

E. 80%

174. Researchers are evaluating a new diagnostic test for detecting breast cancer. The gold standard comparison is mammography plus biopsy. The study results are presented below:

New Diagnostic Test	Positive mammogram & biopsy	Negative mammogram & biopsy
Test positive	95	20
Test negative	5	180

What is the specificity of the new test?

A. 60.0%

B. 82.6%

C. 90.0%

D. 95.0%

E. 97.3%

175. Researchers conduct a study to determine whether the presence of 3 metabolite biomarkers, (taurine, Palmitoyl-l-carnitine, and proline) levels can detect early lung cancer. In the study, 300 individuals (100 with lung cancer and 200 healthy controls) are tested. Combination of 3 metabolites present in 93 lung cancer patients and 5 of the healthy controls. Presence of combination of 3 metabolite biomarkers is considered a positive test for early lung cancer. Which of the following values best represents the specificity of this test?

A. 2.5%

B. 7.0%

C. 50.0%

D. 93.0%

E. 97.5%

176. A clinical trial investigates whether presence of Placenta Growth Factor (PlGF) can serve as an indicator of preeclampsia in a study of 600 individuals (200 pre-eclampsia and 400 healthy controls). The study shows that 168 of the pre-eclampsia patients and 60 of the healthy controls have sFlt-1/PlGF ratio higher than 24.96 ng/ml. sFlt-1/PlGF ratio higher than 24.96 ng/ml. is considered a positive test for pre-eclampsia. Which of the following values best represents the specificity of this test?

   A. 15%

   B. 25%

   C. 60%

   D. 84%

   E. 85%

177. Congenital hypothyroidism is a condition in which a baby is born without the ability to produce normal levels of thyroid hormone. If left untreated, it can lead to developmental delays, growth failure, and intellectual disability. Early detection through newborn screening allows for early treatment, preventing these complications. The condition affects approximately 1 in 4,000 newborns. For screening newborns, the most important goal is to detect every possible case. As a result, the test should prioritize having a high:

   A. Cut off value

   B. Number of true negatives

   C. Positive predictive value

   D. Sensitivity

   E. Specificity

178. Phenylketonuria (PKU) is a metabolic disorder that causes an inability to break down phenylalanine, leading to toxic buildup and potential brain damage. Newborn screening for PKU is a well-established practice that allows early dietary interventions, significantly improving outcomes. The condition affects approximately 1 in 10,000 newborns. Given the potential severe consequences of missing a diagnosis, the screening test should be designed to maximize:

   A. Negative predictive value

   B. Positive predictive value

    C.   Sensitivity

    D.   Specificity

    E.   Validity

179. The standard test for diagnosing disease Z has a specificity of 85%. A research team seeks to improve the specificity and develop a new test. They perform a study on a random sample from the population, and the results are shown below:

New Test	Patients with disease	Patients without disease
Test positive	150	50
Test negative	20	200

Based on these results, have the researchers achieved their goal?

A.   Cannot be determined because the prevalence of disease Z is not provided

B.   No, the researchers' new test has about 5% lower specificity than the standard test

C.   No, the specificity of the new test is nearly the same as the standard test

D.   Yes, the researchers achieved an increase in specificity of about 3%

E.   Yes, the researchers achieved an increase in specificity of about 8%

180. The sensitivity of the standard test to detect disease W is 77%. A group of developers wants to create a new test with higher sensitivity for disease W. They conduct a study, and the results are displayed below:

New Test	Patients with disease	Patients without disease
Test positive	210	90
Test negative	30	410

Have the researchers reached their goal?

A.   Cannot be determined because the prevalence of disease W is not provided

B.   No, the researchers' new test has about 7% lower specificity than the standard test

   C. No, the new test achieves nearly the same specificity as the standard test

   D. Yes, the researchers increased sensitivity by about 5%

   E. Yes, the researchers increased sensitivity by about 10%

181. Carbohydrate antigen 19-9 (CA19-9) is evaluated to be used as a marker for the early detection of pancreatic cancer among at-risk individuals. A threshold value of ≥37 U/mL in the test yields a sensitivity of 81% and a specificity of 90%. Which of the following conclusions about the test results is correct?

   A. Based on a cut point of ≥37 U/mL, 81% of patients without pancreatic cancer will be correctly identified.

   B. Based on a cut point of ≥37 U/mL, 10% of patients with pancreatic cancer will be incorrectly identified.

   C. Based on a cut point of ≥37 U/mL, 81% of patients with pancreatic cancer will be correctly identified.

   D. Based on a cut point of ≥37 U/mL /mL, 19% of patients with pancreatic cancer will be correctly identified.

   E. Based on a cut point of ≥37 U/mL /mL, 90% of patients with pancreatic cancer will be incorrectly identified.

182. A clinical trial examines the diagnostic accuracy of a skin test for predicting allergic reactions to specific food allergens in paediatric patients. A test value ≥3.0 mm is found to have a sensitivity of 58% and a specificity of 85% for predicting allergic reactions. Which of the following conclusions about the study results is correct?

   A. Based on a cut point of ≥3.0 mm, 42% of paediatric patients with allergies will be correctly identified.

   B. Based on a cut point of ≥3.0 mm, 15% of paediatric patients without allergies will be incorrectly identified.

   C. Based on a cut point of ≥3.0 mm, 58% of paediatric patients without allergies will be correctly identified.

   D. Based on a cut point of ≥3.0 mm, 85% of paediatric patients with allergies will be incorrectly identified.

   E. Based on a cut point of ≥3.0 mm, 85% of paediatric patients with allergies will be correctly identified.

183. A new blood test for diagnosing hepatitis C is being evaluated and compared to the gold standard of PCR testing. A total of 1,200 individuals from a high-risk population are included in the study. The results are presented below:

PCR Test	Viral culture positive	Viral culture negative	Total
Test positive	200	50	250
Test negative	30	920	950
Total	230	970	1200

Which of the following represents the positive predictive value of the test under study?

A. 200/230

B. 200/250

C. 230/1200

D. 920/950

E. 920/970

184. A new urinary dipstick test for diagnosing urinary tract infections (UTIs) is being compared to the gold standard of urine culture. A study is conducted with 500 subjects from a population with a high prevalence of UTIs. The study results are summarized below:

Urine dipstick test	Urine culture positive	Urine culture negative	Total
Test positive	70	30	100
Test negative	20	380	400
Total	90	410	500

What is the positive predictive value of the test under study?

A. 70/90

B. 70/100

C. 90/500

D. 380/400

E. 380/410

185. An OB-GYN uses ultrasound to diagnose breast cancer in a population of 10,000 patients, where the prevalence of breast cancer is 1%. The test has a sensitivity of 83% and a specificity of 34%. What is the probability that a patient with a positive test result actually has breast cancer?

   A.   83 / (83+17)

   B.   83 / (83+6534)

   C.   3366 / (17+3366)

   D.   3366 / (6534+3366)

   E.   6434 / (6534+3366)

186. A haematologist uses serum protein electrophoresis (SPEP) to detect multiple myeloma in a population of 2,000 people. The prevalence of multiple myeloma in this population is 1%. The sensitivity of the test is 71% and the specificity is 83%. What is the likelihood that a person with a positive test result actually has hepatitis B?

   A.   58 / (58++142)

   B.   142 / (58+142)

   C.   142 / (142+306)

   D.   1494 / (58+1494)

   E.   1494 / (306+1494)

187. A research team develops a new rapid test to identify viral pneumonia in patients with respiratory symptoms. After evaluating the test, they record the following data:

	Viral Pneumonia		Total
	Present	Not Present	
Test Positive	80	40	120
Test Negative	20	160	180
Total	100	200	300

Which of the following is the likelihood that a patient with a negative test really has viral pneumonia?

   A.   0.33

   B.   0.40

C. 0.67

D. 0.80

E. 0.89

188. Researchers are investigating the accuracy of a new rapid test for identifying patients with malaria. Their results are as follows:

	Malaria		Total
	Present	Not Present	
Test Positive	80	30	110
Test Negative	20	120	140
Total	100	150	250

Which of the following is the likelihood that a patient with a negative test does not have malaria?

A. 0.60

B. 0.75

C. 0.80

D. 0.86

E. 0.93

189. A 65-year-old woman visits a cardiology clinic due to concerns about shortness of breath and chest pain. The physician decides to use a coronary computed tomography angiography CCTA test to rule out coronary artery disease (CAD). Her test result is negative. A study evaluating CCTA in a sample of 1000 individuals aged ≥60, in which the prevalence of CAD is 20%, reveals a specificity of 90% and a sensitivity of 85%. Assuming this patient's pretest probability of having CAD is equivalent to the disease prevalence in the study population, what is the probability that this patient truly does not have coronary artery disease?

A. 68%

B. 72%

C. 85%

D. 90%

E. 96%

190. A 55-year-old woman with a family history of breast cancer is screened for breast cancer using ultrasound. The result of the test turned out to be negative. A study evaluating test ultrasound in a sample of 400 individuals aged ≥50 with similar risk factors, where the prevalence of breast cancer is 25%, demonstrates a specificity of 95% and a sensitivity of 85%. Assuming this patient's pretest probability of having breast cancer is equivalent to the disease prevalence in the study population, what is the probability that this patient truly does not have breast cancer?

    A. 25%

    B. 71%

    C. 75%

    D. 85%

    E. 95%

191. A 62-year-old woman with a history of obesity and smoking presents with a chronic cough. Alpha-1-antitrypsin deficiency (AAT) was tested to this patient. In a recent study, the performance of alpha-1-antitrypsin deficiency compared to spirometry, a gold standard diagnosis of COPD was as follows:

	COPD present	COPD absent
AAT deficient	240	160
AAT not deficient	60	440

The patient is not AAT deficient. Assuming her pre-test probability is equivalent to the prevalence of COPD in the study, what is the probability that the patient does not have COPD?

    A. 60.0%

    B. 73.3%

    C. 80.0%

    D. 88.0%

    E. 90.0%

192. A 50-year-old man with a history of alcohol use presents with abdominal pain and jaundice. Magnetic resonance elastography (MRE) was used to diagnose cirrhosis. The performance of MRE, compared to liver biopsy, which is the gold standard diagnosis of cirrhosis, is summarized as follows:

Magnetic resonance elastography	cirrhosis present	cirrhosis absent
MRE positive	175	25
MRE negative	75	225

The patient receives a positive result on MRE. Assuming his pre-test probability is equivalent to the prevalence of cirrhosis in the study, what is the probability that the patient has cirrhosis?

A. 35.0%

B. 70.0%

C. 75.0%

D. 87.5%

E. 90.0%

193. A new diagnostic test, Shield, detects DNA particles in the bloodstream released by cancer cells. It is being evaluated for its ability to detect colorectal carcinoma at an early stage. The test has a sensitivity of 83% and a specificity of 90% when compared to colonoscopy. The test is applied to two groups: one in Japan, where 36.6 out of 100,000 people have colorectal cancer, and one in India, where 4.9 out of 100,000 people have the disease. Which of the following is the most accurate statement regarding this test?

A. The negative predictive value of the test is lower in the Japanese population.

B. The positive predictive value of the test is higher in the Japanese population.

C. Sensitivity of the test is higher in the Japanese population

D. Specificity of the test is higher in the Indian population

E. The test is not reliable in the Indian population

194. For early detection of lung cancer, the presence of three metabolite biomarkers (taurine, palmitoyl-L-carnitine, and proline) has a sensitivity of 94.4% and a specificity of 97.7% compared to PET scans and biopsies. The test is used in two different populations: a population in Brazil, where 15 out of 100,000 people have lung cancer, and a population in China, where 40 out of 100,000 people have lung cancer. Which of the following statements is most accurate regarding this test?

A. Negative predictive value of the test is lower in the Brazil population

B. Positive predictive value of the test is lower in the Brazil population

C. Sensitivity of the test is higher in the Chinese population

D. Specificity of the test is higher in the Chinese population

E. The test is not reliable in the Brazil population

195. A diagnostic test for obstructive sleep apnea (OSA) is used in a population of 800 individuals aged ≥40. The test has a sensitivity of 90% and a specificity of 85%. The test is then utilized in 2 different populations of individuals of the same age: population 1 has a prevalence of OSA of 12%, and population 2 has a prevalence of OSA of 35%. Which of the following best describes how the negative predictive values (NPV) and positive predictive values (PPV) from populations 1 and 2 relate to each other?

A. PPV in population 1 < PPV population 2; NPV in population 1 < NPV population 2;

B. PPV in population 1 < PPV population 2; NPV in population 1 > NPV population 2

C. PPV in population 1 > PPV population 2; NPV in population 1 < NPV population 2

D. PPV in population 1 > PPV population 2; NPV in population 1 > NPV population 2;

E. PPV and NPV are the same for both population

196. A new test for detecting pancreatic cancer in individuals aged ≥ 60 with a smoking history has a sensitivity of 88% and specificity of 91%. The test is used in two populations: population 1 with a 20% cancer prevalence, and population 2 with a 40% prevalence. Which of the following best describes how the negative predictive values (NPV) and the positive predictive values (PPV) from populations 1 and 2 relate to each other?

A. NPV in population 1 < NPV population 2; PPV in population 1 < PPV population 2

B. NPV in population 1 < NPV population 2; PPV in population 1 > PPV population 2

C. NPV in population 1 > NPV population 2; PPV in population 1 < PPV population 2

D. NPV in population 1 > NPV population 2; PPV in population 1 > PPV population 2

E. A difference in prevalence has no impact on NPV or PPV.

197. Researchers are evaluating Circulating tumor DNA (ctDNA) to diagnose early stages of breast cancer. The presence of ctDNA was assessed in plasma samples, and is being trialled in two groups with different breast cancer prevalence rates. The goal is to assess how well the test performs across both groups by comparing diagnostic parameters. Which of the following performance measures is most likely to vary between the two populations?

A. Negative likelihood ratio

B. Positive likelihood ratio

C. Positive predictive value

D. Sensitivity

E. Specificity

198. A study is being conducted to develop a new test for detecting endometriosis from serum biomarkers and clinical variables. Two test populations, one with a high prevalence of endometriosis and another with a low prevalence, are selected for evaluation. The researchers plan to analyze the test's diagnostic performance across both populations. Which of the following test parameters is most likely to differ between the two groups?

    A. Negative likelihood ratio

    B. Positive likelihood ratio

    C. Positive predictive value

    D. Sensitivity

    E. Specificity

199. A 60-year-old man with a family history of prostate cancer undergoes prostate-specific antigen (PSA) testing. The PSA level comes back within normal limits. He asks his physician, "Given my family history, what are the chances that I really do not have prostate cancer?" Which of the following diagnostic test characteristics would best address the patient's concern?

    A. Accuracy

    B. Negative predictive value

    C. Positive predictive value

    D. Sensitivity

    E. Specificity

200. A 50-year-old woman with a 30-pack-year smoking history undergoes a low-dose CT scan of the chest as part of lung cancer screening. The results come back negative for any suspicious lesions. The patient asks, "Does this mean I definitely do not have lung cancer?" Which of the following test parameters would provide the most useful information to answer her question?

    A. Negative predictive value

    B. Positive predictive value

    C. Precision

    D. Sensitivity

    E. Specificity

201. Researchers evaluate 5 imaging techniques for diagnosing early-stage lung cancer, assessing each for sensitivity, specificity, and area under the curve (AUC). Which technique is the most accurate?

Imaging technique	Sensitivity (%)	Specificity (%)	AUC
1	55.0	77.0	0.680
2	60.0	65.0	0.700
3	70.0	82.0	0.800
4	85.0	88.0	0.910
5	92.0	60.0	0.780

A. 1

B. 2

C. 3

D. 4

E. 5

202. A study evaluates 5 tumor markers for detecting colorectal cancer in asymptomatic individuals, assessing sensitivity, specificity, and area under the curve (AUC).

Tumour markers	Sensitivity (%)	Specificity (%)	AUC
1	47.0	80.0	0.620
2	88.0	65.0	0.820
3	75.0	70.0	0.770
4	60.0	75.0	0.750
5	78.5	85	0.870

Which marker is the most accurate?

A. 1

B. 2

C. 3

D. 4

E. 5

203. A novel enzyme assay, GNS90, is tested for its accuracy in diagnosing severe liver fibrosis. The enzyme concentration (measured in IU/L) is elevated in patients with liver fibrosis. Results from 180 healthy individuals and 160 patients with severe fibrosis are analysed, and sensitivity and specificity were calculated using a cutoff of 100 IU/L (dashed vertical line). If the researchers had used a higher cutoff indicated by a solid vertical line at 120 IU/L, which of the following would most likely be observed?

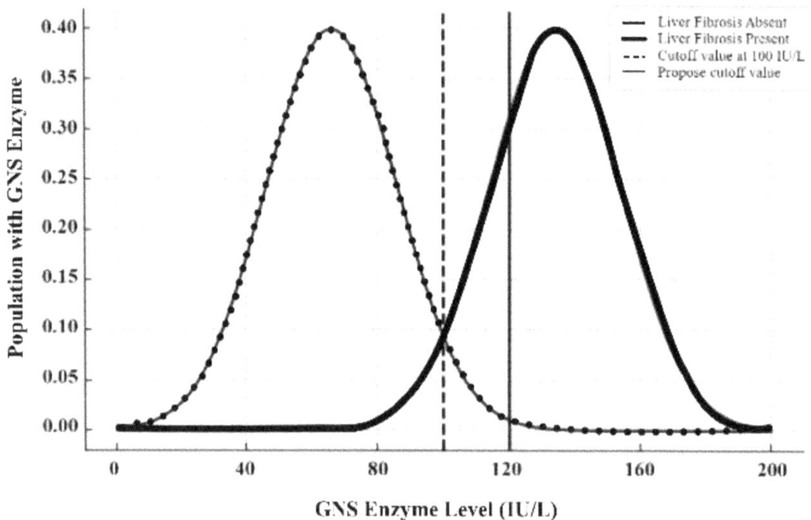

A. Higher number of false negatives

B. Higher positive predictive value

C. Lower number of true negatives

D. Higher sensitivity

E. Lower specificity

204. Carbohydrate antigen 19-9 (CA19-9), is being evaluated for the detection of early-stage pancreatic cancer. The concentration of CA19-9 (measured in U/mL) is found to be elevated in patients with confirmed pancreatic cancer. The test results from 250 volunteers ("healthy") and 220 patients with biopsy-proven lung cancer ("diseased") are shown in a graph similar to the one provided. The researchers calculated the sensitivity and specificity of CA19-9 using a cutoff of 37 U/mL (solid vertical line). If they had instead used a lower cutoff as indicated by a dashed vertical line at 10 U/mL, which of the following would most likely occur?

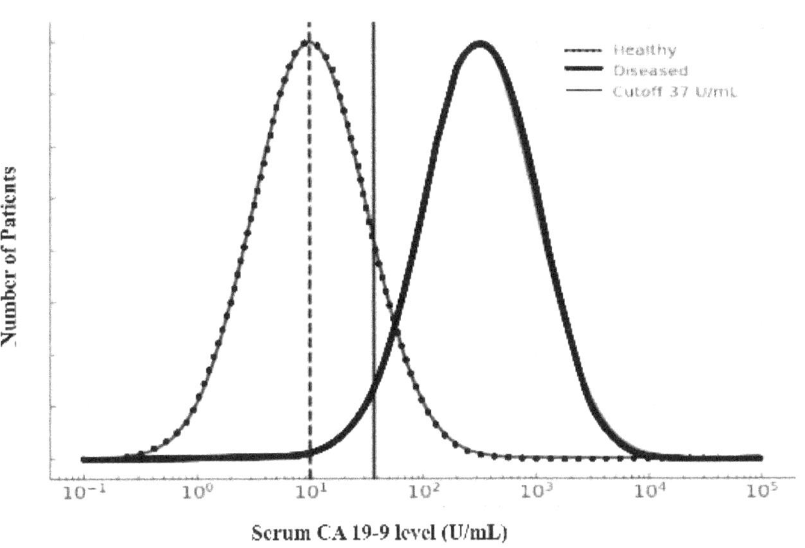

A. Higher number of false negatives

B. Higher positive predictive value

C. Higher sensitivity

D. Lower number of false positives

E. Lower number of true positives

205. A novel liver enzyme assay is being studied for its utility in diagnosing cirrhosis in patients with chronic liver disease. A sample of 350 individuals is stratified into two groups: those with a history of hepatitis B infection and those without. Enzyme levels are measured in both groups, and liver biopsies are used to confirm cirrhosis.

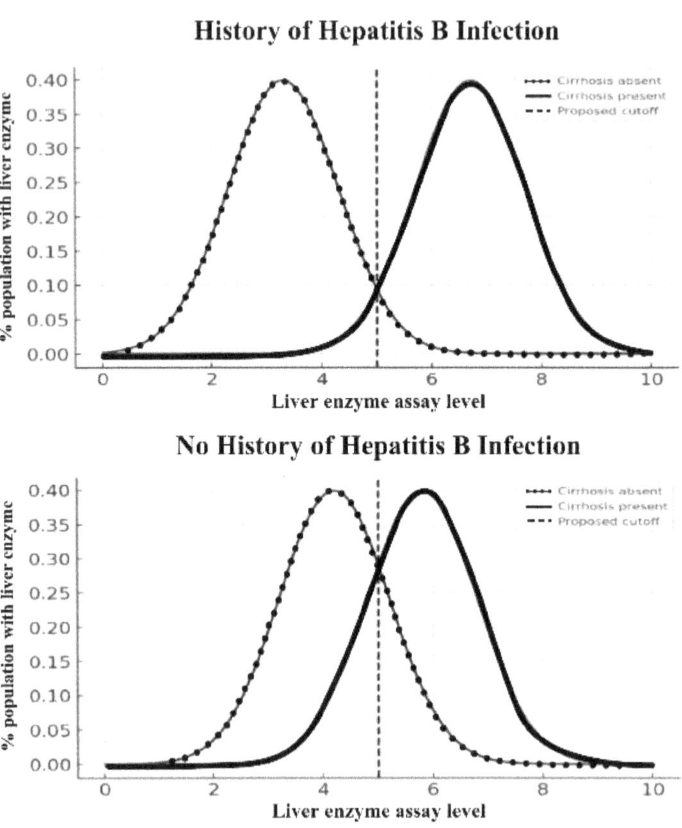

The graph on the top shows the distribution of enzyme levels in patients with a history of hepatitis B infection, while the graph on the bottom shows the distribution in those without a history of hepatitis B infection. The proposed cutoff value for the enzyme assay is indicated. Use of the enzyme marker in patients with a history of hepatitis B infection, compared with those without, is associated with which of the following?

A. Higher sensitivity and higher specificity

B. Higher sensitivity and lower specificity

C. Higher sensitivity and same specificity

D. Lower sensitivity and higher specificity

E. Lower sensitivity and lower specificity

F. Lower sensitivity and unchanged specificity

G. Unchanged sensitivity and unchanged specificity

206. A novel diagnostic marker is being evaluated for detecting breast cancer in women undergoing routine screening. A sample of 600 women is split into two groups based on the presence or absence of hormone receptor positivity. Serum levels of the marker are obtained, and mammography results confirm their disease status.

Hormone Receptor Positive

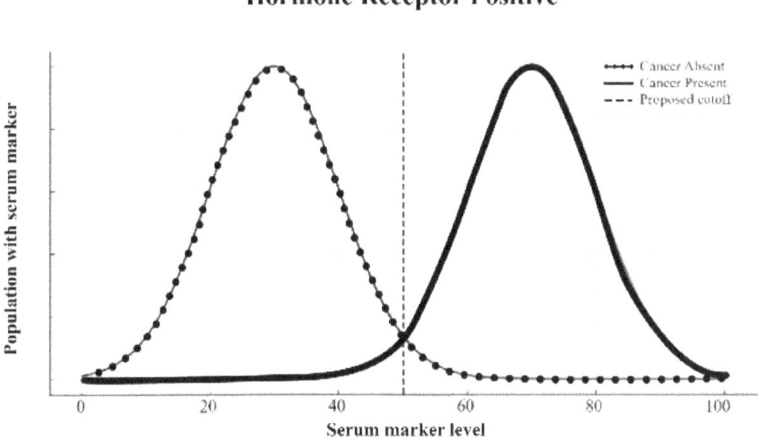

Hormone Receptor Negative

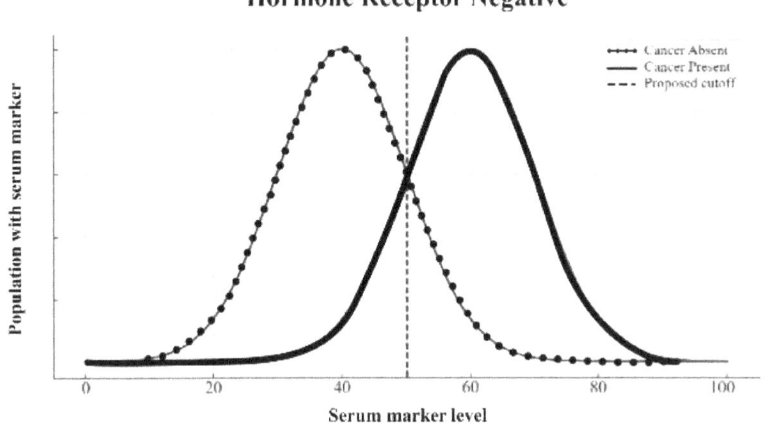

The graph on the top represents the distribution of marker levels in women with hormone receptor-positive breast cancer, and the graph on the bottom represents the distribution in those with hormone receptor-negative breast cancer. The proposed cutoff value for the serum marker is shown. Use of the marker in hormone receptor-negative women, compared with hormone receptor-positive women, is associated with which of the following?

A. Higher sensitivity and higher specificity

B. Higher sensitivity and lower specificity

C. Higher sensitivity and same specificity

D. Lower sensitivity and higher specificity

E. Lower sensitivity and lower specificity

F. Lower sensitivity and unchanged specificity

G. Unchanged sensitivity and unchanged specificity

CHAPTER 8

207. A clinical trial is conducted to investigate the effectiveness of an early mobility protocol for stroke patients in intensive care unit. 50 patients are randomized to either the new therapy group or a control group with standard rehabilitation (25 in each group). After 6 weeks, improvement in mobility scores is observed in both groups, with the early mobility protocol group showing a slightly higher improvement. However, the difference is not statistically significant (p = 0.18). The researchers conclude that the new therapy is not superior. What is the most likely explanation for these findings?

A. Confounding

B. Insufficient statistical power

C. Lead-time bias

D. Recall bias

E. Selection bias

208. A randomized controlled trial is performed to assess the impact of azithromycin preschool children with wheeze. 50 children were randomized to receive either five days of azithromycin or placebo. Primary outcome was time to resolution of respiratory symptoms after treatment initiation. The treatment groups had similar demographics and clinical parameters at baseline. Median time to resolution of respiratory symptoms was four days for both treatment arms (interquartile range (IQR) 3,6; p = 0.28) The researchers conclude that the azithromycin has no effect on time to resolution of symptoms for preschool children with wheeze. Which of the following best explains the study's results?

A. Ecologic fallacy

B. Information bias

C. Insufficient statistical power

D. Measurement error

E. Selection bias

209. Researchers evaluated the weight reduction effects of semaglutide on obese patients with type 2 diabetes. They reported a 5.9 kg difference in weight loss (p = 0.09) between the semaglutide group and the control group, concluding that the new treatment did not significantly reduce weight. However, a subsequent study with a much larger sample size found a significant reduction in weight (difference in mean weight loss = 6.1 kg, p = 0.02). What was the most likely issue with the first study?

A. Confounding bias

B. Insufficient power

C. Lead-time bias

D. Researcher bias

E. Selection bias

210. A small-scale study is conducted to investigate the effect of daily exercise on reducing the risk of hypertension. The researchers find that the relative risk of hypertension among individuals who exercise regularly is 0.90 (p = 0.06), and they conclude that the effect is not statistically significant. Later, a larger study confirms a statistically significant reduction in hypertension risk with regular exercise (RR = 0.88, p = 0.01). Which of the following is the most likely explanation for the lack of significance in the first study?

    A. Measurement error

    B. Misclassification bias

    C. Poor follow-up

    D. Recall bias

    E. Sample size

211. A case-control study is conducted to assess the relationship between vitamin D deficiency and multiple sclerosis (MS). Cases (patients with MS) are recruited from specialized MS clinics, while controls (without MS) are recruited from a general population health survey. The study finds a significant association between low vitamin D levels and increased risk of MS (odds ratio = 2.4; 95% CI = 1.8-3.0). Which bias is most likely affecting the validity of the study?

    A. Detection bias

    B. Lead-time bias

    C. Misclassification bias

    D. Recall bias

    E. Selection bias

212. A clinical trial investigates the effectiveness of a new diabetes medication in reducing averse cardiovascular accident (CVA). Participants are recruited from clinics specializing in diabetes care, and a majority are highly motivated to participate in the trial. The study finds that the medication significantly reduces the risk of CVA in the study population. Which of the following bias is most likely to limit the generalizability of the study's results?

    A. Confounding bias

    B. Information bias

C. Observer bias

D. Recall bias

E. Selection bias

213. A cohort study investigates the association between the use of a certain herbal supplement and the development of hypertension. Participants are asked to report their use of the supplement at the beginning of the study, but no further follow-up is done to confirm continued use. The study concludes that supplement users have a 2.5-fold higher risk of developing hypertension. Which of the following is most likely to affect the validity of this study?

A. Confounding bias

B. Lead-time bias

C. Misclassification bias

D. Recall bias

E. Selection bias

214. A study is performed to determine the relationship between a high-sodium diet and the risk of heart disease. Researchers classify participants' sodium intake based on a single dietary questionnaire. The study reports a significant association between high sodium intake and heart disease. Which of the following is most likely to threaten the validity of these findings?

A. Healthy worker bias

B. Misclassification bias

C. Observer bias

D. Recall bias

E. Referral bias

215. A study seeks to determine whether high caffeine consumption during pregnancy is linked to preterm birth. Researchers interview women who recently gave birth, asking about their caffeine intake during pregnancy. Women who experienced preterm delivery report higher caffeine consumption compared to those who delivered at full term. Which type of bias is this study most likely to encounter?

    A. Confounding bias

    B. Detection bias

    C. Observer bias

    D. Recall bias

    E. Selection bias

216. A public health researcher conducts a case-control study to examine the link between air pollution and lung cancer. Individuals diagnosed with lung cancer are asked about their long-term exposure to air pollution, and the same is asked of healthy controls. Lung cancer patients are more likely to report higher exposure to pollution compared to the control group. What type of bias is most likely influencing this study?

    A. Lead-time bias

    B. Measurement bias

    C. Observer bias

    D. Recall bias

    E. Selection bias

217. A researcher is investigating the association between dietary habits and the risk of developing breast cancer. Mothers of women diagnosed with breast cancer are asked about their dietary intake during their daughters' childhoods. The study finds that mothers of daughters with breast cancer report lower consumption of fruits and vegetables than mothers of daughters without breast cancer. Which type of bias is most likely to affect the validity of this study?

    A. Allocation bias

    B. Detection bias

C. Observer bias

D. Recall bias

E. Selection bias

218. In a study investigating the link between fever during pregnancy and the risk of autism, researchers interviewed mothers of children diagnosed with autism and compared their history of fever during pregnancy to that of mothers of neurotypical children. The results showed that mothers of children with autism reported significantly more frequent instances of fever during pregnancy. What type of bias is most likely affecting the study results?

A. Confounding bias

B. Measurement error

C. Observer bias

D. Recall bias

E. Selection bias

219. A case-control study explores the relationship between sleeping in the prone position and the risk of sudden infant death syndrome (SIDS). Mothers are interviewed about their baby's sleeping posture; mothers of infants who died from SID as cases and mothers of healthy infants as control. The study finds that SIDS cases are more likely to involve prone sleeping. What bias is likely to affect the validity of this study?

A. Allocation bias

B. Measurement bias

C. Observer bias

D. Recall bias

E. Selection bias

220. Researchers evaluate a new educational program to improve asthma management in children. Teachers are asked to assess the students' asthma symptoms before and after the program. The results indicate that symptoms improved significantly according to the teachers' reports. However, it is later revealed that the teachers were aware of which students participated in the program. Which type of bias is most likely affecting the study's findings?

   A. Confounding

   B. Lead-time bias

   C. Observer bias

   D. Recall bias

   E. Selection bias

221. A clinical trial assesses the efficacy of a new antidepressant, with multiple psychiatrists evaluating patients' symptoms using a standardized rating scale. It is found that psychiatrists who are enthusiastic about the new drug report greater improvement in symptoms compared to those who are neutral. What is the most likely reason for this different in reporting?

   A. Confounding

   B. Measurement error

   C. Observer bias

   D. Recall bias

   E. Selection bias

222. A clinical trial aims to test gepirone, a drug for major depressive disorder. The trial involves 300 patients, randomly assigned to take either the drug or a placebo for 12 weeks. Neither the patients nor the doctors who evaluate the outcome are aware of which group is taking the actual drug. This study design helps to prevent:

   A. Attrition bias

   B. Lead-time bias

   C. Observer bias

   D. Response bias

   E. Selection bias

223. In a research study to determine the effect of a cognitive-behavioural therapy (CBT) program on anxiety, 500 participants are enrolled and divided randomly into two groups: one receiving the therapy and the other receiving no intervention. The therapists who deliver the intervention are aware of the assignments, but the researchers assessing the outcomes are blinded to group allocation. This design is primarily aimed at reducing:

    A. Ascertainment bias

    B. Confounding bias

    C. Measurement error

    D. Observer bias

    E. Recall bias

224. A workplace wellness program aims to assess the physical activity levels of employees. Pedometers are distributed to participants to track their daily step counts. After a few weeks, researchers notice that employees are significantly more active compared to baseline. The increase in activity is likely influenced by which of the following?

    A. Berkson's bias

    B. Hawthorne effect

    C. Recall bias

    D. Measurement bias

    E. Misclassification bias

225. A team of researchers is investigating how frequently nurses check patients' vital signs during night shifts. Initially, nurses are unaware that their activities are being monitored. However, after they are informed about the observation, the frequency of vital sign checks increases. What is the most likely explanation for this change in behaviour?

    A. Hawthorne effect

    B. Lead-time bias

    C. Observer bias

    D. Pygmalion effect

    E. Selection bias

226. Researchers introduce a new diagnostic tool for detecting Alzheimer's disease at an earlier stage. Patients diagnosed with this new tool appear to live 6 months longer than those diagnosed with the conventional methods. However, the total number of deaths due to Alzheimer's remains unchanged between the two groups at the 18-month follow-up. What is the most likely cause for the apparent increase in survival time?

    A.   Confounding

    B.   Lead-time bias

    C.   Length-time bias

    D.   Recall bias

    E.   Selection bias

227. A new blood test for early detection of pancreatic cancer is introduced in a clinical trial. Patients who are diagnosed through this test appear to survive 5 months longer compared to those diagnosed through standard imaging. However, at 1-year follow-up, both groups show the same overall survival rate. Which of the following most likely explains the results of this study?

    A.   Confounding

    B.   Lead-time bias

    C.   Length-time bias

    D.   Observer bias

    E.   Selection bias

228. A 10-year cohort study is conducted to determine the effect of daily physical activity on the risk of developing type 2 diabetes. Participants are categorized based on the duration of consistent physical activity: those active for less than 4 years, those active for 4-8 years, and those active for more than 8 years. The study finds that participants who were physically active for more than 8 years had a significantly lower risk of developing type 2 diabetes (relative risk = 0.60, $p < 0.01$) compared to those active for less than 4 years (relative risk = 0.95, $p = 0.42$). The study results were adjusted to account for initial differences in healthy behaviours and overall health. What is the most likely explanation for the reduction in diabetes risk over time?

A. Accumulation effect

B. Lead-time bias

C. Observer bias

D. Misclassification bias

E. Selection bias

229. A prospective study examines the relationship between long-term calcium supplement use and the risk of fracture in postmenopausal women. Women are categorized into three groups: those who used calcium supplements for less than 2 years, those who used them for 2-5 years, and those who used them for more than 5 years. The study finds that women who used calcium supplements for more than 5 years had a significantly lower risk of fracture (relative risk = 0.65, $p < 0.01$) compared to women who used them for less than 2 years (relative risk = 0.98, $p = 0.40$). Which factor most likely accounts for this reduced risk?

A. Accumulation effect

B. Confounding bias

C. Lead-time bias

D. Observer bias

E. Recall bias

230. A randomized clinical trial is conducted to evaluate the effectiveness of Glucose-dependent insulinotropic polypeptide (GIP),a new oral hypoglycemic drug for patients with poorly controlled type 2 diabetes. After obtaining informed consent, eligible participants are randomly assigned, using a computer-generated sequence, to either receive the new drug or a placebo. Both groups continue to receive their standard diabetes management. The random assignment to treatment arms is intended to primarily control which of the following?

A. Confounding

B. Effect modification

C. Observer bias

D. Recall bias

E. Selection bias

231. Investigators are conducting a study on the association between exercise and the development of hypertension. They select a group of individuals with hypertension and a control group of individuals without hypertension. Both groups are matched on age, gender, and body mass index (BMI) to reduce variability between groups. This matching process is intended to address which of the following potential issues?

A. Ascertainment bias

B. Confounding

C. Observer bias

D. Recall bias

E. Selection bias

232. A group of scientists is investigating the relationship between oral contraceptive use and the risk of stroke. They interview a group of women with stroke and a control group of women who do not have stroke. The controls are matched with the cases on age, race, and family history of cardiovascular accidents. This matching technique is intended to minimize the impact of which of the following?

A. Confounding

B. Information bias

C. Lead-time bias

D. Observer bias

E. Selection bias

233. When assigning patients to treatment and control groups, ensuring proper randomization is crucial to prevent the influence of external variables on the study outcomes. In this study, which of the following types of additional information would be most useful for assessing the success of randomization?

A. Annual stroke rates

B. Baseline patient characteristics

C. Patient compliance chart

D. Patient follow-up rates

E. Subgroup analysis tables

234. A case-control study was conducted to assess the relationship between a high-fat diet and colon cancer. The crude analysis showed a significant association between the dietary exposure and the outcome, with an odds ratio of 3.8 (95% confidence interval: 2.5 - 5.2). Physical activity level was considered as a potential confounder of the association. Which of the following properties of physical activity is essential for it to be considered a confounder?

A. It should be evenly distributed among those with and without a high-fat diet

B. It should be highly prevalent in the population of interest

C. It should be observed only in individuals with a high-fat diet

D. It should be related to a high-fat diet

E. It should not be related to colon cancer

235. A study explores the association between hormone replacement therapy (HRT) and breast cancer risk in postmenopausal women. The initial analysis shows a relative risk (RR) of 1.6 with a p-value of 0.04. The researchers stratify the subjects by body mass index (BMI) and find the following:

Group	RR	P-value
BMI < 25	0.98	0.91
BMI ≥ 25	1.02	0.95

The difference between the overall results and the stratified results is best explained by which of the following?

A. Ascertainment bias

B. Confounding

C. Effect modification

D. Measurement bias

E. Meta-analysis

F. Observer bias

236. A prospective cohort study investigates the relationship between the use of oral contraceptives (OC) and the incidence of myocardial infarction (MI) in women. The initial results suggest a relative risk (RR) of 2.0 with a p-value of 0.01. However, after stratifying the data by smoking status, the researchers find:

Group	RR	P-value
Smokers	1.02	0.92
Non-smokers	1.01	0.90

The discrepancy between the overall results and the stratified results is best explained by which of the following?

A. Allocation Bias

B. Berkson's Bias

C. Confounding

D. Detection Bias

E. Effect modification

F. Recall bias

237. A study evaluates the impact of a high-protein diet on weight loss. Among individuals under the age of 40, the diet is associated with significant weight loss (mean difference = 5 kg, p-value = 0.01). However, in individuals over 40, the same diet has no significant effect on weight loss (mean difference = 0.5 kg, p-value = 0.80). Which of the following best describes this phenomenon?

A. Confounding

B. Detection bias

C. Effect modification

D. Lead-time bias

E. Selection bias

238. A trial is conducted to assess the risk of myocardial infarction (MI) with the use of a new cholesterol-lowering medication. In patients with a family history of MI, the drug significantly reduces the risk (RR = 0.70, p-value = 0.02). However, in patients without a family history of MI, the drug has no effect on risk (RR = 1.05, p-value = 0.85). What term best describes this interaction between family history and the drug's effect?

    A. Confounding

    B. Effect modification

    C. Length-time bias

    D. Observer bias

    E. Recall bias

239. Researchers are testing the efficacy of a behavioural therapy program for smoking cessation. In a randomized trial, 180 smokers were randomly assigned to either the therapy group (n = 90) or a control group receiving standard care (n = 90). Participants were followed for 1 year, during which they were asked to attend weekly counselling sessions. However, 10 participants in the therapy group and 5 in the control group missed several sessions. The researchers decide to use intention-to-treat analysis to evaluate the results. How should the data from participants who missed therapy sessions be analysed?

    A. Adjust the analysis only for the therapy group

    B. Analyse participants based on the number of sessions they attended

    C. Conduct separate analysis of the 15 who missed the sessions and 165 who attended the sessions

    D. Include only participants who attended all sessions

    E. Keep all 15 who missed the sessions in their respective groups for analysis

240. A clinical trial is evaluating a new physical rehabilitation program for stroke recovery. Two hundred stroke patients were randomized: one group received the new rehabilitation program (n = 100) and the other, standard care (n = 100). The study protocol involved daily therapy sessions over a 4-month period. Some patients in both groups did not complete all the sessions due to scheduling conflicts or health reasons. The researchers opt for intention-to-treat analysis. What is the most appropriate way to analyse the data for patients who did not complete the full course of therapy?

A. Analyse according to the original group assignments

B. Analyse based on the therapy actually received

C. Exclude all who did not complete the full course of therapy from the analysis

D. Exclude only patients from the standard care group

E. Include only patients who completed all sessions according to the protocol

ANSWER KEY

Chapter 1

1. A	7. B	13. A	19. A
2. D	8. C	14. C	20. B
3. C	9. A	15. D	
4. C	10. A	16. C	
5. B	11. E	17. C	
6. B	12. D	18. D	

Chapter 2

21. D	24. D	27. C	30. F
22. C	25. A	28. A	
23. D	26. B	29. E	

Chapter 3

31. D	35. D	39. C	43. D
32. C	36. B	40. C	44. A
33. D	37. B	41. D	45. E
34. E	38. B	42. D	

Chapter 4

46. A	49. B	52. B	55. C
47. A	50. B	53. KB	56. B
48. B	51. A	54. D	57. E

58. E	65. B	72. D	79. B
59. D	66. B	73. E	80. E
60. E	67. B	74. A	81. C
61. D	68. C	75. D	82. F
62. E	69. C	76. D	83. A
63. D	70. D	77. C	84. C
64. B	71. D	78. F	

Chapter 5

85. C	95. D	105. B	115. D
86. E	96. D	106. B	116. C
87. E	97. C	107. B	117. D
88. E	98. D	108. E	118. D
89. C	99. E	109. C	119. C
90. C	100. D	110. D	120. B
91. E	101. D	111. B	121. E
92. E	102. D	112. D	122. B
93. E	103. B	113. D	123. A
94. C	104. B	114. E	

Chapter 6

124. C	134. B	144. D	154. E
125. E	135. E	145. E	155. C
126. B	136. E	146. C	156. A
127. C	137. D	147. D	157. B
128. E	138. C	148. B	158. A
129. A	139. A	149. A	159. C
130. B	140. A	150. B	160. D
131. B	141. A	151. E	161. C
132. D	142. A	152. A	162. E
133. B	143. A	153. C	

Chapter 7

163. A	174. C	185. B	196. C
164. B	175. E	186. C	197. C
165. D	176. E	187. E	198. C
166. E	177. D	188. D	199. B
167. C	178. C	189. E	200. A
168. B	179. B	190. E	201. D
169. B	180. E	191. D	202. E
170. E	181. C	192. D	203. A
171. C	182. B	193. B	204. C
172. D	183. B	194. B	205. A
173. E	184. B	195. B	206. E

Chapter 8

207. B	216. D	225. A	234. D
208. C	217. D	226. B	235. B
209. B	218. D	227. B	236. C
210. E	219. D	228. A	237. C
211. E	220. C	229. A	238. B
212. E	221. C	230. A	239. E
213. C	222. C	231. B	240. A
214. B	223. D	232. A	
215. D	224. B	233. B	

9 7 9 8 8 9 6 9 9 7 7 3 3